OUT OF THE BLUES

OUT OF THE BLUES

A new approach to helping women overcome depression

Zita Annette Weber PhD

mg

Published by
Margaret Gee
PO Box 221, Double Bay NSW 1360, Australia
Tel: (02) 9365 3266 Fax: (02) 9365 3168

First published 2000

Copyright © Zita Annette Weber, 2000

All rights reserved.
No part of this publication may be reproduced, stored in a retrieval system,
or transmitted in any form or by any means, electronic, mechanical, photocopying,
recorded, or otherwise, without the prior written permission
of the copyright owner.

National Library of Australia Cataloguing-in-Publication entry
Weber, Zita Annette
Out of the blues:
a new approach to helping women overcome depression

ISBN 1 875574 37 9

Design and print management
Reno Design Group, Sydney R19135
Designer Graham Rendoth
Printing Griffin Press Pty Limited, Netley
Distribution Gary Allen Pty Ltd, Sydney
Publishing manager Sardine Waters

'And then the woman saw that the tree was good for food, and that it was pleasant to the eyes, and a tree to be desired to make one wise, she took of the fruit thereof, and did eat, and gave also unto her husband with her; and he did eat.'
Genesis 3:6

'Unto the woman he said, I will greatly multiply thy sorrow and they conception; in sorrow thou shalt bring forth children; and thy desire shall be to thy husband, and he shall rule over thee.'
Genesis 3:16

'Pandora sat in the dying light. She knew that she, woman, would be blamed for this monstrous happening, so she sealed a memory within herself which could be discovered by women of the future. It was the memory of feeling at one with a great feminine presence who filled her with belief in herself. Remembering this power in her own body, she had lifted the great cornucopia of life, and poured hope into the world.'
Lindel Barker-Revell

DEDICATION

*This book is dedicated to two wonderful women:
Margaret Gee and Kimberley Cameron.
Thank you for providing support and encouragement.*

CONTENTS

	Author's Thanks	8
	Acknowledgements	9
	Introduction	10
1	Are You Depressed?	13
2	Female Vulnerabilities	31
3	Images of Women	53
4	The Challenge of Relationships	81
5	Trouble in the Teen Years	108
6	Birth Blues	124
7	A Baby Maybe	143
8	When a Mother Loses a Child	163
9	Vulnerable Points and Processes	186
10	Taking Control of Your Life	232
	Coda: Hope – The Legacy of Pandora	245

AUTHOR'S THANKS

I would like to thank all the people who, over the years, have contributed one way or another to my work.

Many women shared their experiences and their stories in the spirit of generosity and courage. Clients who had the courage to tell all; interview respondents who wanted to tell their story in order to make a difference; and group participants who were willing to undertake tasks and exercises which not only helped them, but added to my understanding of women's depression: you all are part of the following pages.

The ideas and work of my colleagues and other professionals have guided and informed my research and added to the richness of my direct work with women, both individually and collectively.

My special thanks go to Kimberley Cameron for keeping the faith and introducing me to my agent and publisher, Margaret Gee. Margaret's enthusiasm has made this book possible. Thank you both for believing in me.

Again, thank you John, for encouraging me and giving me the space to write.

ACKNOWLEDGEMENTS

The author acknowledges the work of the following authors, whose scales, exercises and quizzes have been adapted in the search for suitable and relevant tasks to use with women experiencing depression:
- Tennant and Andrews, 1976
- Boyce, 1987
- Tanner and Ball, 1989
- Montgomery and Morris, 1989

INTRODUCTION

Depression has been described as a universal experience and a normal human experience. No-one is immune to a case of the 'blues'. Research studies in different countries and cultures and across all social classes show a similar frequency of depression.

The late Lady Diana, The Princess of Wales, spoke about her depression and her self-destructive behaviour. She told Panorama's Martin Bashir in her much publicised 1995 interview:

> *'When no-one listens to you, or you feel no-one's listening to you, all sorts of things start to happen... You have so much pain inside yourself that you try to hurt yourself on the outside... Yes, I did inflict pain on myself. I didn't like myself. I was ashamed because I couldn't cope with the pressures.'*

Not being able to cope with pressures is a common cause for depression. Lady Diana received, in the first week after she spoke out, 6,000 letters from women who identified with her and who, like her, had experienced desperate unhappiness in their lives. These women have low self-esteem, poor self-value and their sense of disappointment, shame and guilt result in self-attacks.

While depression is no respecter of colour, creed or class, it does seem to affect women more. Women are twice as likely than men to experience an episode of depression. According to academic and psychologist Dr Leslie Brody: *'Men are about four times more likely to commit acts of violence than are women, while women are about twice as likely to become depressed as men.'* Women also are more likely to seek help.

In this book, you will be introduced to ideas and theories about depression. You also will meet women who share their experience of

INTRODUCTION

depression and their ways of coping. Their stories show the ways out, through and around depression. There are no simple answers or cures for depression. But there is information and knowledge.

Every woman has a story. Each story imparts some information, some knowledge. In 1597, Francis Bacon wrote: *'Knowledge is power'*.

You are invited on a journey in the following pages. A journey to gain more knowledge and to understand depression. Understanding depression leads to a sense of empowerment. At the end of this book, you will be in a better position to cope with depression.

You'll meet women who've battled with depression caused by a number of different stresses and strains of everyday living. Some women will talk about their depression which is related to relationship difficulties and breakdown, others will share their depressive feelings about their roles as wives, mothers and workers, and sometimes the balancing act involved in having all three roles. Still other women will tell us about their diet-related depression, their baby-blues, their age-related depression and the depression linked with infertility and other traumatic life events. Traumatic life events include losing a parent, a spouse, finding out your husband is having an affair – with another man, and the bitter-sweet pain of being 'the other woman'.

Then there are those women who experience mood swings and recurring depressive episodes. There are many reasons why women get depressed. Understanding some of these and learning how other women have won through leads to a sense of hope.

By becoming aware of what helps and hinders your mood and sense of well-being, you will develop better strategies to make changes in your life. You will gain a sense of satisfaction and personal power when you realise your skills and strategies can make a difference. You can control your depression and improve your mood.

Finding your way through the maze can lead to a more productive life. Women who have been able to 'pick up the pieces' offer insights into how you can restart your life.

Taking control of your life is your aim. Taking control of your life means you have empowered yourself. It might have started with Eve, but women's vulnerability to depression can be transformed by understanding how you can use hope to overcome your vulnerability.

Pandora, who was Greek mythology's Eve found hope and let it loose into the world. From Eve to Pandora, women can experience vulnerability and they can experience hope. It's up to you to explore your vulnerability and find your own version of hope.

1
ARE YOU DEPRESSED?

> *'I am rather blue today, all the meaning of fate falling on me over the weekend in the form of a nasty sinus cold and a very painful slipped disc in my back... also two rejections of poems and stories from the disdainful **New Yorker**.'*
>
> SYLVIA PLATH, [Letters Home]

Sylvia Plath was no stranger to depression. Born on October 27, 1932 in Boston's Memorial Hospital, Sylvia's genius became apparent early in life. When she was 14, she surprised her high school English teacher, Wilbury Crockett, with poems she had written. Prizes at school and praise at home were threatened by emotions from within. Sylvia was a young woman aware that she was vulnerable and that the world could hurt her.

The poem she showed Mr Crockett was titled *I Thought That I Could Not Be Hurt* and it shows a sensitivity that was to haunt Sylvia all her life.

I thought that I could not be hurt;
I thought that I must surely be
impervious to suffering –
immune to mental pain
or agony.

My world was warm with April sun
my thoughts were spangled green and gold;
my soul filled up with joy, yet felt
the sharp, sweet pain that only joy
can hold...

Then, suddenly my world turned gray,
and darkness wiped aside my joy.
A dull and aching void was left
where careless hands had reached out to
destroy

my silver web of happiness...

Throughout her life, Sylvia's personal hell was managed through her work. She dealt with her depression by writing constantly about herself – defining herself and managing the outside world through her literary material which reflected her personal experience. She sustained her spirit until she couldn't fight her fragility anymore.

Depression is a widely felt emotion. It describes a debilitating emotional condition. It is a feeling of being pressed down by the world. There is one powerful message. While some of us are unusually vulnerable to depression, none of us is immune. Even if we escape the experience personally, we will eventually encounter a family member, friend or colleague who feels bleak about themselves and the future.

We often avoid using the word. Instead, words like 'the blues', 'feeling down', 'feeling low', 'being out of sorts' have become popular ways of expressing the experience of depression. Depression is hard to define and hard to predict. It can strike anyone at any time and at any age. Often there is a great deal of shame attached to feeling like you're not coping. And fear that others will notice. As Lady Diana said, 'I was ashamed because I couldn't cope with the pressures.' The language that people use to describe the experience of depression provides strong clues about the darkness and isolation that envelopes them.

THE LANGUAGE OF DEPRESSION

Depression covers a spectrum. The English language has been used richly to describe these depressive feelings. Colours like black and blue are used frequently, and body parts, like the heart, are linked to our moods. Many depressed people will talk about falling into a pit, or being in a long, dark tunnel. Often the idea of hope is represented by 'the light at the end of the tunnel'.

Every kind of metaphor imaginable has been used to conjure up the experience of depression: to suffer a broken heart, to be sick at heart, go into the doldrums, to be crestfallen, cut up, to feel flat, to be downcast, be blue. So endemic is depression that there's a form of music simply called 'the blues'. We may not talk about it openly, but we can listen to someone singing about their 'blues'.

DEPRESSION AS CRISIS

Depression can be viewed as a crisis. Crises are life problems which demand more than your usual routine coping. A crisis provides an opportunity to learn more about yourself and your view of the world. In the Chinese language, the word 'crisis' has two representations, one is the character meaning danger, the other the character meaning opportunity. Such an opportunity enables you to further develop your coping strategies.

For some women, depression provides the opportunity to rebuild a life based on more understanding of themselves and an acceptance of their emotional lives. One woman called depression, 'the special gift' that had turned her life around. Some women see their depression as the strongest factor in determining the person they had become.

Until people see a checklist of the symptoms of depression they may think that depression means feeling so awful you can't function and so low that you feel suicidal. Some women report going to work every day, feeling like work projects are insurmountable, having little energy and no desire to socialise, sleeping restlessly, but not recognising that they are depressed. One woman said, *'I thought you had to be suicidal to be depressed. I was hanging in there – okay, life was miserable, but I wasn't considering killing myself'*. Then she saw a checklist and decided to get some professional help.

Some women, it seems, adjust to a low-grade chronic depression and don't realise that they are depressed. Such a situation can endure for months or years until something happens to alert the woman to her plight. In such cases, the full impact of the depression hits the woman when there is some shift, however subtle, in her way of being. Perhaps she has always felt off-colour, a little down but believed that her low spirits were part of everyday life. Then she read something, saw something or talked to someone and realised she was depressed. Her discovery can be in the form of a sudden realisation or a dawning one in which the reality slowly starts to fall into place.

Other women put up a good front and defend themselves against their depression – at least publicly. They may feel depressed – utterly hopeless and despairing of the future and still appear to be functioning reasonably well. It might be the case that their denial of their feelings is easier when they take pills or drink alcohol. The gap between the surface picture and reality might be a significant one. One client told me she was the *'Mistress of keeping my real feelings well out of sight and pretending life was a breeze'*. All the while, her own personal hell was kept at bay with practised pretense and a fondness for cocktails and sleeping pills. But her mask began to slip and her crutches proved inadequate and eventually she became desperate enough to seek help.

MILD, MODERATE AND SEVERE DEPRESSION

Depressive episodes can be mild, moderate or severe. Sometimes depression can be experienced as initially mild, then become moderate and even severe. The reverse is also true. Progression from one state to another is common. A severely depressed woman is someone who is unable to look after herself. Her general health suffers and she may be at risk of self-injury or suicide. She may be lethargic or extremely agitated.

For some women, depression is not progressive. It is rather more static, with some women reporting a chronic low level or mild depression over a number of years. On the other hand, if a depression becomes severe enough, it might be labelled a 'clinical depression'. This term means that the depression is serious enough to require treatment.

Depression is best viewed as ranging along a continuum. This continuum is in terms of depth and severity, as well as the extent to which physical, emotional, psychological and social functioning is impaired. It is difficult, in reality, to identify one point where a depression becomes 'clinical'.

Signs and symptoms of depression: A checklist
1. Depressed mood, feeling sad, low, blue, despondent, hopeless, gloomy
2. Loss of energy, fatigue, lethargy
3. Anxiety
4. Changes in appetite
5. Sleep disturbance
6. Bodily complaints, such as headaches, stomach pain, for which there is no medical explanation
7. Loss of sex drive
8. Changes in posture, grooming, speech
9. Loss of interest in usual work and social activities
10. Diminished ability to think or concentrate with mixed-up thoughts and slower thinking
11. Feelings of worthlessness, self-reproach, guilt and shame
12. Feelings of helplessness
13. Fall in self-esteem
14. Thoughts of death and suicide

Very rarely do depressed women experience only one of the signs described. Most women report multiple symptoms. She usually experiences depressed mood plus four or five other symptoms.

Often women visit their doctor, believing something is physically wrong with them. Physicians report that a large number of depressed patients present themselves in the first instance with 'vague physical aches and pains' – symptoms such as chronic headaches, neck and back pain, stomach pains and sleep disturbances. One physician told me that in such cases he always asks the patient: 'How are your spirits?', as a way of prompting the patient to share her feelings.

Maggie Scarf, in her book **Unfinished Business**, writes about what she considered 'those bizarre statistics on women and depression'. She was surprised to find that, *'For every male diagnosed as suffering from depression, the head count was anywhere from two to six times as many females'*. Surprising the statistics certainly are. They are also compelling and beg some explanation. For the fact is, that women from adolescence onwards, are far more vulnerable to depression than men. In every subsequent stage of the life-cycle, women are more vulnerable. Men and women are never equal when it comes to depression.

Contrary to popular belief, women become depressed long before the onset of menopausal chemistry becomes the standard explanation for women's greater vulnerability. In my practice and research, I have found higher numbers of women reporting their experiences of depression. These women have come from every social class and represent every age group.

WHAT WOMEN SAY

'I remember going into the doldrums just before my 40th birthday. I wrote in my journal, "I'm closer to 40 than 39. I want time to stop. I have no practice at being 40". But I turned 40 anyway and I was depressed for about six months, until I got a grip on things and realised it wasn't the end of my life as I know it. But I do think it's hard for women in this society. You know, 40 is such a big hurdle.'

Eva, 43

'When I was depressed, everything seemed futile. There was no purpose to anything in life. Everything was hopeless. I thought this feeling would never end. Sometimes I felt I couldn't face the day.'

Corinne, 34

'I used to get very depressed when I was at high school. I used to keep a 'blues diary' and I wrote down all my dark thoughts and feelings... I wasn't in the right clique and I didn't make the sports teams, so I hid a lot in the library. I guess I had a low opinion of myself.'

Melissa, 20

'I know now that all my life, my dose of the blues was related to one thing only – men. I couldn't get it right with men and relationships. It took me until I was 35 to settle down with a caring man who valued me for myself, and not because I was supposed to be a Barbie. I think men are the cause of a lot of depression among women. Especially younger women.'

Leigh, 38

'When I'm depressed I can't sleep, eat or rest – I'm fidgety and I cry a lot. My depression is usually related to some sort of disappointment. Last time it was being fired, the time before it was a relationship split-up.'

Karen, 28

'I've only been depressed really badly once. It was after my mother died. We had a very close relationship. The depression affected my whole body. I felt paralysed, like parts of my body didn't work. I had terrible indigestion, I couldn't think straight I was so distraught with the loss.'

Blythe, 32

'Shortly after I had a miscarriage, I plunged into the depths of despair. I felt all wrong. I got agoraphobic and I ate all the time. I thought I was a failure. I felt lousy, ugly and evil. I felt so alone. I couldn't be consoled, although people around me tried hard.'

Lyn, 25

'I felt so miserable I thought I'd fallen down a deep pit. I sometimes thought I was clawing my way out but bits of the sides would break off in my hands and I'd fall even further. I remember wondering how I'd get up from the bottom of the pit, climb out and get on with the rest of my life.'

Joan, 55

'When my doctor told me I was going through the change of life, I sort of felt that life was over for me. I had all these silly ideas about life not being worth living. But, as it happened, my symptoms were not that bad and soon I realised that it wasn't the end for me. I remember walking down the street thinking, 'what a lot of fuss about nothing', life was still interesting and I threw myself into it wholeheartedly.'

Maree, 53

'I was very down when my kids were younger. You know, it's exhausting looking after three kids under five. I didn't have enough support and some days I thought I was going mad. I was irritable, moody, teary and constantly tired.'

Tricia, 36

'After my second baby was born, I had a dose of the baby-blues. I was very down, and what made it worse was that my husband wasn't very supportive. He wanted just as much attention as before and was always too tired to help me with anything. He's a pretty selfish man, and now he had two other little people to compete with. I've always said, I have three children. Finally I managed to get out of the depression, I guess I owe it to a neighbour, who's like a mother to me.'
Judy, 29

'I thought I had a marriage made in heaven – until my husband walked out on me and the two kids. He'd been seeing another woman for two years. I thought I'd die – I felt so rejected and alone. I got very depressed for about a year.'
Jenny, 34

These women have had a bout of the blues. Their words convey the despair and hopelessness of their experience. But as Gloria Steinem found, depression offers an opportunity to redefine your life. Redefining your life can mean making small and large changes. It is possible that such changes are hard to make without the spark offered by a depressive experience.

DEPRESSION: AN OPPORTUNITY FOR GROWTH

You'll recall the earlier reference to depression as crisis. A crisis can offer the opportunity to make changes.

In ***Revolution From Within: A Book of Self-Esteem***, Gloria Steinem candidly talks about her experience of and exposure to depression from an early age. Steinem recalls her bedridden mother who had nervous breakdowns and severe depressions for most of Steinem's childhood. Her foodaholic, three-hundred pound father, who left when she was 10, also suffered from depressions from time to time, when his business dreams were dashed.

Steinem describes emotional and physical losses which probably created a vulnerability to depression. During her teenage years, Steinem developed body image problems, which are so pervasive today. Steinem describes herself as *'a big, plump, vulnerable girl... growing up in an isolated family whose food addictions and body image'* she took on board. Two decades later, as a 34 year old freelance journalist, she became active in the then growing women's movement. In her words, *'Feminism saved my life'.*

However, the legacy of childhood experiences and social conditioning are difficult to challenge. Steinem opted for a variation on the theme. She did not become a wife and mother, but she spent 20 years of her life as an activist and advocate for the women's movement. Like other women, Steinem had learned to take better care of others than herself. At 50, she faced head-on the vulnerabilities and stresses that ageing brings in a youth-centered society. She was exhausted and found that she was under tremendous pressure which lead to *'a burnout and erosion of self so deep that outcroppings of a scared 16-year-old began to show through'.*

Finding some solace in a relationship and facing a bout with breast cancer around the same time brought Steinem to the crossroads. She admitted that depression had been a backdrop in her life. Setting aside her belief that therapy was for other people, not for her, she found a woman therapist.

Steinem admits to having become *'lonely and depressed... and then more lonely and depressed'.* She was motivated to improve life by the very despair she felt. She wrote, *'...there's something to be said for hitting bottom: as with swimming, it may be the only way to propel oneself back up again.'* Steinem's inner exploration allowed her to make the connections between her caretaking role for her invalid mother and the selfless caretaking of others that is expected of women in our society. While her commitment to the women's movement nurtured the needs of many others, she was not taking care of her inner needs. Inattention to yourself can lead to stresses and strains and a chronic feeling of depression.

Positive outcomes can come from an experience of depression. Gloria Steinem was not alone with her feelings of depression, nor was she the first person to recognise that facing depression can change your life – and in a positive way.

There is an undeniable positive side to depression. This positive side is best seen when you are on the other side of the depressive experience.

While you are in the grips of the experience, it's hard to see any of the pain and agony as positive, or potentially growth-producing.

In **Care of the Soul**, Thomas Moore, a therapist, writes: 'Depression grants the gift of experience not as a literal fact but as an attitude toward yourself. You get a sense of having lived through something, of being older and wiser. You know that life is suffering and that knowledge makes a difference'.

WHAT ABOUT POST-TRAUMATIC STRESS DISORDER (PTSD) – IS IT LINKED TO DEPRESSION?

Post-traumatic stress disorder is not the same as depression. However, a woman suffering from PTSD may experience depression. Traumatic events such as being the victim of a violent crime or any personal assault or witnessing such events are extremely stressful. PTSD usually starts within six months of the traumatic event. Women report feeling depressed and they might also have thoughts of suicide. There may be a reliving of the trauma through flashbacks or dreams.

A NOTE ABOUT DEPRESSION AND MANIA

So far, only what is called 'unipolar' depression has been discussed. This means that the woman suffers only from depression. Those women who suffer from both depression and mania are said to have a 'bipolar' disorder or manic-depression.

Is bipolar disorder more prevalent among women? A review of the literature shows that while depression is more common among women than men, depression and mania affect women and men about equally. Manic-depression is less common, and affects about one in 200 people. The term 'mania' describes an increased mental and physical activity. A woman who experiences manic-depression has excessive mood swings from deep depression to euphoria. At times, it can make the person lose touch with reality, but inbetween, there may be periods of total normality.

Women who have experienced manic-depression speak about the adrenaline rush of the manic phase making them feel high, allowing them to thrive on very little sleep, having them believe life is terrific, no challenge is too great and often, giving them a supreme sense of feeling they are great or significant or specially chosen. Many women experience a fast flow of ideas and a pressure to speak – because thoughts are moving rapidly, and everything is very significant, there is a sense of urgency – a pressure to communicate at once.

Sometimes there is increased sexual activity and a woman may become less discriminating about the people she has sex with. Some women report an increased insensitivity to other people, even women who can normally empathise with others become very self-centered. Coupled with an increased self-preoccupation is a lack of insight or self-criticism.

Many women feel more religious or spiritual. These feelings may be very powerful and a woman may feel she has been chosen to be the next Virgin Mary. A sharply reduced sense of danger is part of many manic episodes. Dangerous sports, gambling, foolish business investments and reckless driving can be evident when a woman is manic. Spending lots of money without thinking of or caring about the consequences is also common manic behaviour.

For women who experience manic-depression, the depressive episodes are characterised by symptoms common to depression: lack of energy, a sense of extreme fatigue and hopelessness, lack of concentration, 'worthless' thoughts, feeling irritable, feeling dead emotionally, appetite and sleep disturbances and changes in self-image, with feelings of being ugly, nothing looking right and feelings of guilt.

Rosanna, a 30 year old actress was diagnosed as being manic-depressive about five years ago. She talks of the pleasure and the pain of her condition. She knows her parents have been frightened by her behaviour and sometimes finds herself feeling ashamed for the things others tell her she did when she was manic. She says:

'Being manic feels great. The first time I felt that way, it lasted six months – I felt energetic, creative and confident. Everything was just right. I had heaps of adventures, I fell in love constantly. I acted on impulse – and it felt good.

I stopped balancing my cheque-book, and I bought everything that I saw and wanted – because I knew I was going to win the lottery. I was sleeping maybe three hours and as the weeks went by I got crazier and crazier. I remember convincing a friend to take a drive with me, telling her that I could drive as fast as wanted and we'd be safe.

When I'm manic, it's like there's an extreme clarity and awareness – a little like taking a hallucinogenic drug. We went on that drive and I crashed the car. I still can't understand how we both escaped uninjured – it's a bit eerie, almost as if my feelings of being Superwoman – of not being harmed by anything I did, was true.

I'm horrified and a little ashamed of some of the things I've done and said while manic. Friends tell me I went through a real promiscuous phase. They said I used to walk around radiating love and generosity and flirting with every man in sight. I do remember having sex with a cabdriver, instead of having to pay the fare.

But my worst experience was being in a full-blown manic state when my parents arrived to see me. I was talking very fast, and a lot of gibberish. I was hurling furniture around and saying I had important business to attend to. My parents were horrified to see me eating bits of the manuscript I was studying and tearing up $10 notes because the face on the money offended me. I was in a terrible state, packing and unpacking my bags and prowling around restlessly. But, do you know, that once they got me to the hospital, I remember feeling relieved, thinking, yes, please, let it be over, please turn off the energy, turn off the lights, let me relax.'

Rosanna's description of her mania captures some of the common features of the manic phase: rapid thinking, intense insights, impaired judgement, uncontrollable excitement and a reduced sense of danger.

Manic depression has the potential to disrupt a woman's life. As Rosanna adds, *'And when I'm neither up or down, I'm just like anyone else.'* However, it's the being 'up' and 'down' and dramatically 'crazy' or 'blank' behaviour that follows that causes difficulties in the lives of women afflicted – and those around them.

Two famous names, both actresses suffered from manic-depression. One was Frances Farmer, who describes her ordeal honestly and horrifyingly in her autobiography, ***Will There Really Be a Morning?*** The other was Vivien Leigh of whom Tennessee Williams once said, *'Having known madness, she knew how it was to be drawing close to death'*. Vivien Leigh was a complex woman, a woman of great extremes and excesses. A stage actress who won acclaim for her Juliet, Antigone and Cleopatra, she also received two Oscars for two of the most celebrated roles in film history, Scarlett and Blanche. Vivien Leigh was said to have had an insolence towards life and yet believed, like Blanche, that everyone had a right to magic.

There is a story about how the magic of Vivien Leigh's performance captured the legendary producer Alexander Korda. Sitting in the stalls of the Ambassadors Theatre in May 1935, Korda was to watch Vivien Leigh transcend the expected stereotyped performance as a prostitute. She possessed the kind of magic that made the passionate street girl appear to be a great lady. Or the reverse, that the great lady could be a street girl. Korda is said to have observed a complex duality in Vivien Leigh's personality. When he congratulated her, he was humbled, saying, *'Even a Hungarian can make a mistake'*. Korda was to prove to be right in his assessment of Vivien Leigh's personality, and her acting abilities. Her personality and mesmerising duality would be played out memorably in portrayals of the two sides of the 'dual' woman.

WHAT CAUSES MANIC-DEPRESSION?

Research has not given us any definite conclusions. Some researchers believe there is a genetic predisposition to manic depression, which is triggered off by stress. Others think that it may result from severe emotional damage during early life, which gives the person a very fragile sense of self. Another view is that chemical imbalances in certain parts of the brain can affect moods. It's important to understand that after a period of mania or depression, a person returns to their usual personality without any psychological harm. Often people experience feelings of regret about the damage done to relationships and finances.

Treatment can require mood-stabilizing drugs, antipsychotic drugs, and sometimes ECT (electroconvulsive therapy). Alternative therapies involve managing mood swings by recognising what is likely to be stressful, recognising the onset of mania or depression, learning to relax, maintaining a regular lifestyle, exercising regularly and changing thought patterns to emphasise the positive things in life. Keeping track of life with a diary can be a powerful tool in helping a woman understand how to reflectively meditate. A diary can help put day-to-day events in perspective and give insight.

The idea of keeping a diary or journal to record what's happening in your life – your thoughts and feelings – is a good one. It helps you develop self-understanding. You don't have to write daily entries, only when you feel the need to do so.

UNDERSTANDING YOUR DEPRESSION

Keeping a diary can help you understand your moods. But let's start at the beginning. A good beginning is to be able to rate your mood. The following exercise helps you understand how you might discover more about yourself.

Exercise   Rating your mood department

By keeping track of your moods, you will understand more about yourself. The following scale helps you record your moods.

Instructions
Rate how you are currently feeling on the following nine thoughts and feelings. Place an X on each of the lines at the position on the line where your mood is best reflected.

Eg. I do not feel hungry ————X———————— I feel as hungry as is possible

1. I do not feel sad at all ———————————————— I feel so sad that I can't stand it

2. I get as much pleasure from things as usual ———————————————— I get no pleasure from doing things

3. I look forward to pleasurable events ———————————————— I am unable to look forward to things

4.	I do not feel feel guilty	I feel as guilty as possible
5.	I do not feel unworthy	I feel totally unworthy
6.	I do not feel slowed down physically	I feel completely slowed down physically
7.	My thinking is clear	I find it difficult to think at all
8.	I do not feel anxious	I am as anxious as I have ever been
9.	I have as much energy as usual	I have no energy at all

(Adapted from *Visual Analogue Scale*, Boyce, 1987)

How to use the scale

Complete the scale each week. Compare your results before and after reading this book and learning the skills and strategies you can use.

You may be surprised by your ratings. Perhaps you have never sat down and thought about some of the signs that have been bothering you. By seeing your responses, you can begin to understand how you are affected. And that means you can start working on getting better.

THE DEPRESSIVE CYCLE

Beware the triad of feelings and emotions, behaviour and thinking involved in the depressive experience. It looks like this...

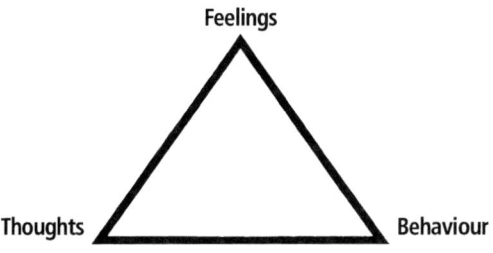

When you feel bad, you are less likely to do things, especially new and different things. You have doubts about your ability to succeed.

When you are successful at something you feel good. You gain confidence. When you feel that you can do something well, you are more likely to try things.

You can visualise this as a feedback loop.

How you feel affects how you think and behave, which affects how you feel, and so on. You are caught up in an interactive system, where each thing affects the others.

When you go into a depressive spiral you believe you have few positive outcomes in your life and you feel depressed. Then, because you're feeling depressed, you do less. Because you're in this mood state, your thoughts become increasingly negative. You then feel even worse and then you do less. And so on.

The depressive or downward spiral looks like this...

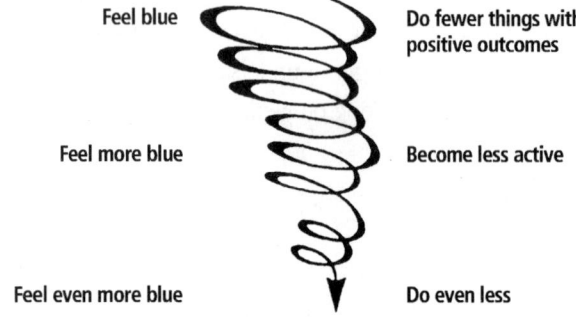

Feel blue	Do fewer things with positive outcomes
Feel more blue	Become less active
Feel even more blue	Do even less

But, a positive spiral is also possible. You have to break the negative cycle and change it.

The first step to take to hook into the positive or upward spiral is to become aware of what you find pleasurable and what activities give you a feeling of accomplishment.

The positive or upward spiral looks like this:

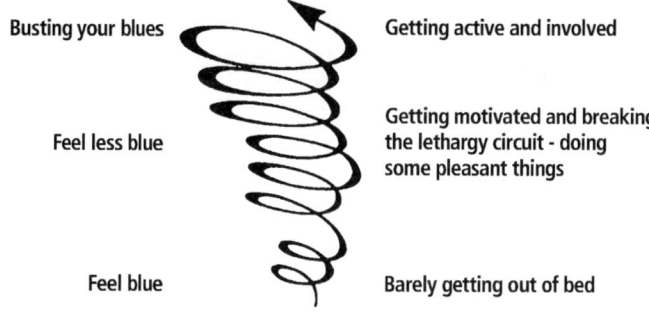

Busting your blues

Feel less blue

Feel blue

Getting active and involved

Getting motivated and breaking the lethargy circuit - doing some pleasant things

Barely getting out of bed

It's important to understand the positive benefits you can achieve from gaining a sense of mastery, of satisfaction in having completed a task. Doing something pleasurable when you're feeling blue is preferable to doing nothing at all.

Complete answers to the statements which follow to gain insight into what you consider as potential pleasant activities.

As you identify activities which give you pleasure, try to include them in your day and your week and look for other activities you might enjoy.

Exercise Looking at what gives you pleasure

Instructions
Select and rank activities according to their satisfying qualities.
- recreational activities enjoyed before the blues
- learning activities enjoyed before the blues
- day trips enjoyed
- things that might be enjoyed if you had no inhibitions
- things previously enjoyed alone
- things previously enjoyed with others
- things that were enjoyed that were free
- things that were enjoyed that cost less than $10.00
- things that were enjoyed when money was no object
- things that could be enjoyed if money were no object
- activities enjoyed at different times of the day, the week, seasonally

Get in touch with pleasurable feelings and activities. It will give you a sense of owning something positive. That's an important step in hooking into the positive spiral.

You have to unlearn old habits. Old habits that stop you from trying something new. Old habits that stop you from being adventurous. Old habits that undermine your confidence.

CIRCLE THIS

Develop the new habit of making an action plan for yourself. Maybe that night course in French culture is the pleasurable activity which you've been putting off for years. Go to a free concert in the park. If walking barefoot on the beach makes you feel good, make the effort to do it. Start doing things that are pleasurable for you. If not today, then maybe next weekend.

Remember the words of Mark Twain: *Habit is habit and is not to be flung out the window, but to be coaxed downstairs a step at a time.*

But coaxed downstairs and out of your life – bad old habits must go! If you want to regain your vitality, you have to be active. Activity is essential to life.

Decide today to get active – Life. Be in it!

2

FEMALE VULNERABILITIES

*Catharine's state of mental depression
lasted throughout December 1829.*

**CATHARINE BEECHER
[A Study in American Domesticity]**

Catharine Beecher is said to have suffered a 'nervous collapse' when her plans for a moral department in her school were refused. Catharine Beecher's life is an early example of the tension between a woman's internal and external worlds. Stress can lead to depression. Catharine's strong sense of self was tempered by the stereotypes through which American society, at that time, viewed her. As a pioneering teacher and writer on moral and religious topics, she became a household name as an avid publicist for women's education. Her *Treatise on Domestic Economy* was a comprehensive guide to all aspects of domestic self-management which would provide women with social influence and a female domain from which to exercise cultural power. It would appear that Catharine was disappointed, stressed and became depressed.

STRESS AND DEPRESSION

Life is full of stresses and strains. That means it can also be full of disappointments and unresolved problems. We all have to deal with our identity, our ambitions and needs while coping with the demands of people and events in our lives. These events can feel like pressures. Sometimes these pressures are obvious and current and sometimes they are 'unfinished business' from the past.

CIRCLE THIS

We all have a store of things in our pasts which we sometimes feel unhappy about. For some women, these things are minor, maybe making a mistake at work, or being jilted. For others they might be more major: a terrible disappointment, being jilted for some women at certain times in their lives will be a major disappointment. Others might include losing a spouse, failure of a business, a geographical move including a new job, which doesn't work out as hoped, children leaving home, illness and bereavement.

Perhaps you think these events are just everyday ordinary occurrences. Of course, you're right. They are. But they can also trigger depression.

WHAT TRIGGERS DEPRESSION?

Your feelings of depression are most likely to arise in times of stress. Triggers for your depression may include social and psychological crises, stressful life events and excessive stress.

SOCIAL AND PSYCHOLOGICAL CRISES

Women move through a predicted series of stages throughout life. Some of these stages are called 'crises' because they test the person's coping style. These crises are life problems which demand more than the usual routine coping. It is useful to view each crisis as providing the opportunity to learn more about yourself. Learning more about yourself leads to better coping skills.

Crises: early, middle and late

The first crisis and test comes with the teenage years, when the most important questions are 'Who am I?' and 'What's it all about?' The teenager experiences a lot of biological and psychological changes and social pressures. Often the result is irritability and depression.

Melissa, a 20 year old college student was depressed during her teenage years. She believed she was unattractive, felt badly about herself and disliked the social pressures around her to be feminine and popular. She said:

'I used to get very depressed when I was at high school. I used to keep a 'blues diary' and I wrote down all my dark thoughts and feelings. I wasn't pretty or cute or anything. And I got branded a 'brain' which is the best way to become unpopular – if you're seen as bright you can't be a feminine girl.

'Anyway, I didn't want to be a Barbie Doll – I just wanted to be taken seriously – but most kids my age were scared of me. I wasn't in the right clique and I didn't make the sports teams, so I hid a lot in the library. I guess I had a low opinion of myself.'

As women move into their 20s and 30s, life becomes more predictable and a routine sets in. However, adjustments that have to be made in the 40s and 50s mean another testing time for coping skills.

With the ageing of the 'baby boomer' generation, there has been more written about the crisis of ageing in youth-dominated society. Fear of the loss of physical health, the readjustment required by retirement and the perceived loss of usefulness are real tests of coping skills. Coming to terms with this crisis means rethinking your place in the world. Your self-esteem might fall rapidly and if you can't adjust to a new and different role, then you can end up feeling depressed.

For some people, especially attractive women, who have been prized for their looks, ageing can be a major crisis and a source of depression.

Susanna, an attractive fortysomething woman, former model, mother and homemaker, found that ageing represented a crisis. She said:

'One of the big things in my life was my image of myself and how I looked was really important to me. I was born lucky – dealt a good hand, if you like. Even as a little girl I was treated like a rare jewel. I had the sort of conventional beauty which is highly valued. I was a natural blonde, with clear deep blue eyes and I was real cute. As I grew up I developed the classic 36-24-36 and because I was 5'8" and leggy, I looked great.

Everyone said I should be a model and that's what I became. I led a charmed

> *life for many years. I had a good husband, who was respected in the legal community, two beautiful boys and my only worries seemed to be how I'd organize my social schedule for the coming week.*
>
> *I felt secure until I was about 38 when I noticed that people didn't stare anymore. I was so used to walking into a room and having people stare at me that when it stopped happening I missed it terribly. People might turn around and look at me now but they don't stare. I lost that power to stop them dead in their tracks at about 38. What's strange is that it didn't happen gradually, it seemed to happen overnight. One day I was being feted and given lots of attention and the next day I was treated like an ordinary person. I missed being special. It was very depressing. And then my husband walked out on me. He found what he called a 'younger version' of me. I went into a very deep depression.'*

Susanna had to recover her sense of self – and redefine herself. She had to work on lifting her self-esteem and thinking differently about herself and her future. She found it a challenge, but she succeeded. She overcame her depression by understanding herself better and coming to terms with different expectations and taking control of her mood – and her future.

Life events and difficulties

Your depression may be triggered by events which involve some change in your daily life. Life events are major changes, like the breaking up of a relationship, starting a new job, financial difficulties, and even having a baby. Even if a life event is pleasant, such as having a baby, there may be great stresses involved, which can trigger depression.

A new baby and the role adjustments for the couple are sources of stress. It's been found that between 10% to 30% of women experience a post-natal depression in the first six months following the birth of their baby.

Cindy, a 28 year old woman and first-time mother became depressed a week after giving birth to her son. Recently, she had coped with a number of life events, including moving to another state, being separated from family, friends and support systems, giving up her full-time work, having to support her husband in his highly pressured new job, and not least, needing to adjust to her new full-time role as a mother. Added to these stresses were her unrealistic expectations of herself. She said:

> 'Now that I'm a mother, I must be totally responsible. I have to be perfect – like my mother was. I feel really terrible, but I can't ask for help because it'll be seen as a sign of weakness. I just have to learn to cope with it all – and get to like it. Sometimes I think I've reached breaking point – I don't have any new friends yet and my husband is preoccupied with his new career. I feel trapped – and once I had ideas about hurting my baby. That frightened me. But, I'm a mother now and I'm going to have to cope. I know that's what my mother would want and I expect myself to live up to her view of me.'

Cindy had to learn to develop more realistic expectations of herself. She had to adjust to her new role and not be concerned with what others might expect of her. She had to learn to think differently about herself and her needs. Cindy overcame her depression by expressing her thoughts and needs and learning to be more realistic about herself, her roles and how other people fitted into her life.

Life events cannot be avoided. But you can learn to reduce the amount of stress they place on you.

Sometimes women get the blues when there is no obvious stressful life event. Their low feelings may be the end result of years of general unhappiness, unresolved conflicts and ongoing relationship difficulties. Sometimes there is a delayed reaction to something that happened in the past – maybe a long time ago.

Does stress cause depression? As we've seen, stressful life events contribute to your mood. But what do we mean by stress?

WHAT IS STRESS?

People speak about being 'stressed out' and we've all heard about 'stressors' in our lives, things like feeling isolated, working too hard, having too little money and failing to meet our own or others' expectations of us.

The word 'stress' is used in a number of ways. First, it can mean the cause of someone's troubles. Secondly, it can mean the troubles themselves. Thirdly, it can mean the impact of these troubles on the troubled. Added to this is the distinction that we have to make between 'good' and 'bad' stress.

'GOOD' STRESS

This is the sort of stress that we feel when we are 'charged up' for a performance event. Ask any sportsperson, actor or student before an exam. They feel charged with adrenalin. Their hearts beat faster, their blood pressure rises, the blood supply is directed to muscles to help them move and their breathing rate increases. You've probably heard this called the 'flight or fight' response. This is a short-term reaction geared to meet a specific need.

'BAD STRESS'

This flight or fight response may be triggered by a psychological threat to your emotional well-being, like a relationship break-up or job loss. But, instead of being a short-term response, it can be extended over a longer period.

People start to feel anxious when this happens. This sort of extended high anxiety can make you feel vulnerable to feeling flat – getting the blues.

WHY CAN SOME PEOPLE COPE WITH MORE STRESS THAN OTHERS?

This is an unknown. What is known is that the level of stress for optimum performance varies from one person to another. The ability to tolerate 'bad stress' also varies considerably. Some people can tolerate and even thrive on high levels of arousal.

Learn to understand which level of stress you're comfortable with and adjust your lifestyle to that comfort zone.

Lifestyle

Take a good look at your lifestyle. We've all heard a lot in the media about the importance of a healthy lifestyle. There's no denying that stress affects a physically unfit woman more than a woman who has paid attention to her body.

Keeping in shape, eating well, not skipping meals and not overworking or partying to excess is the key to a healthy lifestyle. If you don't observe sensible rules of living then feelings of irritability and depression will inevitably follow.

Learn to understand the balance between work and pleasure. Consider your body a temple. Work on your relationships. Give yourself time off to enjoy hobbies. Learn to relax. And, just occasionally, indulge yourself in the luxury of just being.

By completing the following exercise you can see the current stressors in your life.

Exercise Life events questionnaire

If you look at the first column, 'Distress' measures the amount of psychological and emotional stress caused by the event. In the second column 'Life change', you'll find a measure of the magnitude of changes to your routine.

Instructions
Circle any of the following events which you have experienced in the past 12 months.

Event	Distress scalings	Life change scalings
Health		
1. You had a minor illness or injury like one needing a visit to a doctor or a couple days off work	2	2
2. You had a serious illness, injury or operation needing hospitalization or a month or more off work	16	16
3. A close relative had a serious illness (from which they did not die)	16	9
4. You are pregnant (with a wanted pregnancy)	2	26
5. You are pregnant (with an unwanted pregnancy)	33	29
6. You had a stillbirth	40	22
7. You had an abortion or a miscarriage	26	13
8. You had a baby	5	47
9. Your change of life (menopause) began	14	18
10. You adopted a child	4	47
Bereavement		
11. Your husband/partner died	83	79
12. A child of yours died	80	57

13. A close family member died (eg. parent, brother, etc.)	57	27
14. A close family friend or relative died (eg. aunt, uncle, grandmother, cousin etc.)	30	12

Family and social

If you are or were in a permanent relationship...

15. You married	5	59
16. There has been increasing serious arguments with your husband/partner	26	25
17. There has been a marked improvement in the way you and your husband/partner are getting on	2	18
18. You have been separated from your husband/partner for more than a month because of marital difficulties	31	29
19. You have been separated from your husband/partner for more than a month (for reasons other than marital difficulties)	12	15
20. You have got back together again after a separation due to marital difficulties	5	25
21. You began an extramarital affair	14	28
22. Your husband began an extramarital affair	35	28
23. You have been divorced	54	62

If you have children...

24. A child of yours became engaged	2	6
25. A child of yours married with your approval	2	10
26. A child of yours married without your approval	22	16
27. A child of yours left home for reasons other than marriage	11	14
28. A child of yours entered the armed services	9	10

If you are single...

29. You became engaged or began a 'steady' relationship	2	17
30. You broke off your engagement	25	21
31. You broke off a 'steady' relationship	18	18
32. You had increasing arguments or difficulties with your fiance or steady friend	15	13

Friends and relatives

33. A new person came to live in your household (apart from a new baby)	8	20

34. There has been a marked improvement n the way you get on with someone close to you (excluding husband/partner)	1	10
35. You have been separated from someone important to you (other than close family members)	13	13
36. There has been a serious increase in arguments or problems with someone who lives at home (excluding husband/partner)	16	16
37. There have been serious problems with a close friend, neighbour or relative not living at home	10	8

Education

38. You started a course (college, apprenticeship or other occupational training course)	3	16
39. You changed to a different course	5	11
40. You completed your training program	2	27
41. You dropped out of your training program	14	22
42. You studied for, or did, important exams	10	13
43. You failed an important exam	20	18

Work

44. You have been unemployed and seeking work for a month or more	20	22
45. Your own business failed	38	44
46. You were fired	32	34
47. You retired	15	53
48. You were downgraded or demoted at work	20	18
49. You were promoted	2	18
50. You began to have trouble or disagreements with your boss, supervisor or fellow workers	10	9
51. You had a big change in the hours you worked	5	16
52. You had a big change in the people, duties or responsibilities in your work	7	17
53. You started in a completely different type of job	8	24
54. You had vacation for a week or more	1	5

Moving house

55. You moved here from overseas	19	48
56. You moved to a new city	8	26
57. You moved house	4	11

Financial and legal

58. You had moderate financial difficulties	9	10
59. You had a major financial crisis	34	37
60. You are much better off financially	1	23
61. You were involved in a traffic accident that carried serious risk to the health or life of yourself or others	31	22
62. You had minor difficulties with the police or the authorities (which has not required a court appearance)	4	12
63. You had more important problems with the police or authorities (leading to a court appearance)	21	15
64. You had a jail sentence or were in prison	59	72
65. You were involved in a civil law suit (eg. divorce, debt, custody, etc.)	25	21
66. Something you valued or cared for greatly was stolen or lost	9	5

(Adapted from *Life Events Questionnaire*, Tennant and Andrews, 1976)

Scoring

Look to where you have marked an event. Add the number of points under 'Distress' and 'Life Changes' separately.

How to Interpret Your Score

Distress scores	Low	Medium	High
	0 to 10	20 to 30	61 to 200

If you scored between 0 and 10, you have not experienced significant emotional stress in the past 12 months.

Scores between 20 and 30 indicate that you have been exposed to a fair amount of emotional stress.

Scores above 61 suggest you have experienced a significant amount of emotional stress in the past 12 months – possibly enough to lead to a depression.

Life Change scores	Low	Medium	High
	0 to 20	30 to 40	81 to 200

Your level of exposure to life changes has been minimal if you scored between 0 and 20.

If you scored between 30 and 40, you have been exposed to a higher than average number of life changes.

Scores above 81 suggest your life changes have been exceptionally high in the past 12 months.

If you scored highly, be aware that your depression could be related to life events and the difficulties you've encountered in the past 12 months.

WHAT'S SO DEPRESSING ABOUT BEING A WOMAN?

Being a woman means you are two or three times as likely to be depressed as a man. These differences begin early. Studies have found that depression was observed in girls 'definitely more' than in boys. Depending on the statistics used, the number of teenagers who suffer from depression ranges from one in five to one in eleven. Until the teenage years, depression affects boys and girls almost equally. However, after age 12, the rate for girls increases. By the age of 14, girls are twice as likely to be depressed as boys. Women are more vulnerable to depression, but why?

Experts still have difficulty in answering this 'why' question. In fact, there is continuing difficulty in answering 'what causes depression?'. It seems there is no right answer. Often there are multiple factors which lead to a person's vulnerability to depression.

Explanations regarding women's depression range from the biological – 'raging hormones' idea, to the psychological and sociological. Some theories are narrow, while others permit a broader explanation, still others combine factors to form a more complex, life-like picture of the tyranny of depression in many women's lives.

Let's look at the competing explanations about female depression.

A WOMAN'S BODY

Sometimes female depression is explained in terms of biological factors. Maybe the woman has a hereditary predisposition to depression, with a parent or grandparent who was depressed. Perhaps she has a biological depression. This simply means that her depression is caused by an abnormality in the body's chemistry or metabolism, and not by stress or problems in living. Often a woman's raging hormones are blamed. It seems the female endocrine system is more sensitive than that of the male! A hormone is a substance which is excreted directly into the blood by the endocrine gland.

Research is inconsistent about the relationship of hormone levels to depression. This doesn't mean that some women will not have hormone-related depression, but it does mean that it's not the complete answer. Many women's vulnerability to depression increases in the post-natal period, and pre-menstrual tension and oral contraception also have their effect, but only to a very small degree. Contrary to widely-held views, there is good evidence that menopause has little or no effect in increasing rates of depression and pregnancy appears to decrease the risks. Of course, the everyday life stresses and strains around pregnancy and the menopause may provoke vulnerability, but in and of themselves, they have been found to not increase a woman's likelihood of getting depressed.

Take note: Researchers have concluded that genetic and hormonal explanations of higher rates of female depression are not convincing enough. Explanations involving social and psychological factors appear to be more important.

Currently, the biological or more accurately, biochemical explanation of depression is in vogue. These depressions are called 'endogenous' and appear to 'come out of the blue' and for no apparent reason. The British psychiatrist, Anthony Clare believes that many psychiatrists are *'too busy to do more than undertake a cursory examination of their patient's history and mental state'.* Consequently, Clare contends that they *'diagnose an excessive number of depressions as arising 'out of the blue'.*

Research indicates that most depression is what's called 'reactive'. That's to say, the depression comes in reaction to a specific event or situation, one which usually involves a change in life situation. In fact, it's been estimated that up to 75% of all depression is reactive in nature.

WOMEN'S SOCIALISATION

According to one theory, women may be more vulnerable to depression because of the way they have been socialised into the female role. The experiences of our early years are crucial for developing the inner resources and strengths which make us as individuals, more or less vulnerable to depression. Early experiences can affect a woman's functioning and vulnerability in later life.

Without positive early experiences, it might be difficult to have the self-respect, strength and inner resources needed to deal with life's circumstances. One research study found a relationship between early and later life experiences. If you have suffered a childhood loss then it is more likely that a loss in adult life will bring on a depressive experience. The childhood loss that was studied was an actual separation or emotional absence experienced by the child.

This explanation holds true for Andrea, 42, an administrative assistant. She lost her mother at the age of 13 and lost her childhood because her father and two older brothers expected her to assume household responsibilities. Andrea remembers feeling overwhelmed. She also remembers not being allowed to express her distress. Her father's motto was 'you got on with your life.'

'I didn't have a very happy childhood. My mother was sick for a long time before she died. It was painful watching her being so ill. But we weren't encouraged to talk about it, so all these powerful feelings were locked up inside me. It wasn't till years later that I realised why I was so depressed a lot of the time.

'I felt put-upon and devalued by my father and brothers after mom died, but again, I couldn't talk about it to anyone really. Not until much later. I guess I've felt depressed a lot of my adult life because I had lost my mother, whom I adored and I was left with very little – a mean-spirited father and two demanding brothers. And to make things worse, I married a very hard man, who didn't make me feel any better. We didn't have any children and after five years we divorced. It was after the divorce that I went to see a counselor to sort out my life.'

Another woman, Carmen, 44, who works as a personal assistant to a company vice president speaks about how she spent years overcoming the early message she received about not being important in the external world. Today, she comes across as warm and secure, the sort of person you immediately feel you can relate to. She says:

'I come from a migrant family where the boys took pride of place. There were two boys and three of us girls. My parents were very keen for my brothers to have a good education and to 'get ahead' in the world. We girls were given the message that the boys were better than us and that our role in life was to get married, have kids and stay at home playing the good, faithful housewife. In a way, I – and my sisters – were made to believe we were worthless.

'I don't mean our parents set out to do this, but that was the end result of their attitude to the boys and girls in the family. My two sisters bought that message – they're both married, not happily, and one of them is very depressed about never having what she calls 'done anything' with her life. She tells me she's envious of my life. I tell her that I've struggled with depression – trying to overcome that early message – and feeling guilty that I haven't married and done all the right things. My parents were disappointed earlier on, but now I think they're resigned to the fact that I haven't grown up to be the 'good girl' they trained me for. Like I say, I've had bad bouts of depression, but I believe I understand more about myself and I think I've resolved most of my past problems.'

Sometimes, feelings of insignificance or inferiority are reinforced by other aspects of female socialisation. A little girl learns very early on that she should comply, please and give others what they want and expect. As she grows up, the young woman finds she has little sense of what her own needs are. Or she thinks that her own needs are unimportant and unworthy of attention. These feelings may lead to a vague sense of something missing, a feeling of some deprivation. Very often these feelings of 'something missing' are not recognised for what they are. Instead, a woman may find herself feeling depressed.

Diane tells a story in which her early training in feelings of selflessness appears to be linked to her later depression. She is 36 and the mother of two teenagers, a girl aged 15 and a boy, 14. She speaks quickly, with a sense of urgency in conveying her message:

> 'I suppose I learned to be sweet and kind and all those feminine things when I was a child. I had two brothers and they were allowed to be as selfish and rowdy as they liked. I was the only girl and I can remember being told to be a 'little lady' when I was about six. I was supposed to look after my brothers, even though they were older than me – this was the case particularly when we were teenagers.
>
> 'My mother was the same. She was practising what she was preaching. She looked after everyone, and seemed to have no needs of her own. I was always a little jealous that she seemed to care more for my brothers, but I later understood why. Girls are meant to be able to look after themselves and everybody else as well!
>
> 'I've always been careful to not give my own daughter that message. She's allowed to be just as selfish as her brother. I hope she'll grow up with less heartache about all of this. I used to get terribly depressed and I felt as guilty as hell, if I thought I was paying some attention to myself. After all, I was a woman and a mother and had no right to think of myself. It's taken a long time to sort that out.'

Little girls are expected to grow up like their mothers. This means developing a keen sense of the needs of others and placing those needs ahead of their own. To be nurturing and emotionally giving is the lot of a woman.

Perhaps Margaret Mead's words in *Male and Female* still hold some truth:

> 'The small girl learns that if she simply waits, she will some day be a mother; the small boy learns that he is male and that if he is successful in manly deeds some day he will be a man.'

Although the women's movement has made some inroads into this pattern of socialisation, we have a long way to go. There are many young girls still who are brought up in families with traditional gender-role expectations. These girls are taught to be tidy and clean, passive and pretty, coy and attentive to others. They are given curfews and warned about the dangerous world that faces them – 'a man's world' where the only way a woman can advance is to use her 'feminine wiles'. Consequently, these girls are discouraged from developing another part of themselves – an independent, strong, assertive side. Growing up being passive, dependent, fearful, self-sacrificing and subservient is not conducive to good mental health. In fact, qualities such as passivity, dependence, submission form the core components of depression.

Torri is a 19 year old who has suffered from depression over the past five years. She is a good student and in the second year of her university course. Although her academic work is something in which she takes pride, she is despairing much of the time about her future. Torri speaks slowly as if measuring the impact of her words. She is conventionally pretty and tells me she hates being told she is, because it's 'so sexist'. She comments:

'When I was young I was a bit of a tomboy – and a bit loud I guess. My parents disapproved of my being that way – and they made me into what I am today. They've helped me suppress my real self. It's become buried. I'm scared of showing people my real self, because I've learnt that it's bad to be strong and loud. Instead, what you see today is what I've become, rather withdrawn,]
'I started going to counselling about a year ago, and I've had all these insights about myself. I'm working hard on de-programming myself and getting back to my real self. I know if I find that tomboy I might have to face harsh consequences – like rejection by my parents.'

Susan Brownmiller, journalist, author and feminist, claims that gender-conscious parents speak to their girls and boys quite differently from the outset. She writes:

'Mothers and fathers tend to use a higher singsong register with baby girls, a sweet coo of 'Isn't she pretty?' as opposed to a brisk, jovial 'Hey, how's the little feller?' and 'Look at the little guy!' Children are great imitators – how else are they going to learn? – and the process of mimicry in the child helps to set the speech pattern for the adult.'

Brownmiller also suggests that the end product is women speaking 'in feminine' and men speaking 'in masculine'. Women are schooled to speak softly and less often as speech is considered to be an assertive act.

Some 20 years ago, researchers found that gender-stereotyped behaviour in women correlated with low self-esteem, high levels of anxiety and poor emotional adjustment. On the other hand, women who had an 'androgynous' identity (both masculine and feminine characteristics) were found to have good self-esteem and a sense of who they are. They were outgoing, creative and successful professionally. These findings suggest women pay a high price for being 'feminine'. By breaking out of the traditional gender-role expectations and becoming more androgynous, women may be more protected against depression.

If socialisation patterns make women vulnerable to depression, what about psychological factors?

PSYCHOLOGY'S ROLE IN FEMALE VULNERABILITY

Psychologists called Behaviourists believe that depression is the result of a reduction of positive reinforcements in a person's life. A lack of these reinforcers are abundant in many women's lives. As the previous women's quotes tell us, many women find it hard to get positive reinforcers because they've been encouraged to be passive rather than assertive. Often women's roles are unsatisfying and therefore, lacking in positive reinforcement. Many women, to achieve desired aims, have had to depend on covert behaviour – 'feminine wiles' – rather than open and direct communication. This leads to distortions in personal relationships and fewer positive reinforcers for women.

What's called 'learned helplessness' is another behavioural theory. Based on laboratory experiments, this theory suggests that when a person is denied the opportunity to control their environment in their early years, they are more likely to feel a sense of helplessness in adult life. This theory may highlight some of the reasons why women are prone to depression more than men. As the researchers Beck and Greenberg comment:

> *'(Women) are taught that their personal worth and survival depends not on effective responding to life's situations but on physical beauty and appeal to men, i.e. that they have no direct control over the circumstances of their lives.'*

While little boys are still encouraged to take risks, to be heros and to tackle the world, little girls are told they shouldn't get dirty, nor should they take risks. Little girls are still told: 'Don't shout, don't swear, be a good girl' and in brackets we might add: 'Then you might be rewarded with a husband and children'.

Because women typically assume powerless roles, they have fewer opportunities for reversing this tendency of helplessness later in life. Added to this is the suggestion that women have what's been labelled, 'negative attributional style'. Studies have shown that women are more likely than men to attribute their success to luck and serendipity or external factors. On the other hand, women also are more likely to attribute their failures to personal inadequacies. Consequently, women are less likely to expect to succeed in the future and less likely to try.

Elaine, 57, a senior executive, provides a good example of how past lessons influence future endeavours. She is a tall, attractive woman who speaks with authority. However, as she unfolds her story, it's clear that her sense of security is relatively newly found. She says:

> *'It's taken me about 30 years to get over my thinking that my success is simply a matter of 'being in the right place at the right time'. I used to struggle with the idea that I earned my position. This is where I've found male and female thinking very different. Most of the men I know just take it for granted that their success was due them – it had very little to do with outside factors. I felt like my success had everything to do with outside factors for a long time. I couldn't believe I had really been good enough, or competent enough, or anything enough for that matter, to get to the position I'm in.'*

Cognitive psychologists believe that human emotions are the result of what people think or tell themselves. They suggest that depression is caused by negative thoughts and perceptions of yourself, the world and the future. It is believed that a woman's negative view might be related to early experiences such as a loss of a parent or a significant adult in childhood. Also, this theory suggests that women are more bound to their 'internalised oppression' – they see themselves as dependent, helpless and repressed.

Freud and his more modern followers believe that anger and depression are linked. This psychoanalytic explanation of depression puts forward the view that anger turned inward, a frequently 'feminine' pattern, creates depression. Each time a woman denies her feelings, blames herself for others' behaviour, makes excuses for others' inappropriate behaviour, she turns her anger on herself.

The depression that women experience may well hold their anger in check. Their depression may become the repository for all intense emotions, which are 'inappropriate' for a woman to display. After all, depression is socially acceptable, whereas negative feelings are not.

Anita, 49, is a woman who impresses as confident, sure of her path. However for many years she suffered depression. She tells of her chronic depression, throughout her 22 year marriage – and her anger. But she felt guilty about feeling angry, so it was driven underground, and she suffered depression. She says:

> 'After 22 years I was free – free to be myself, my angry, unacceptable, real self. All my marriage, I'd been the 'good' wife, mother, daughter-in-law, sister-in-law etc. etc. I used to take a lot of Valium to get through my life. Sad isn't it? I thought there was something wrong with me – but all along, it was because a part of me was dying and I couldn't express my anger.
>
> 'I felt resentful that I was slowly dying as a person but my ex-husband was a dominating man – an excellent provider and a good man – but not a caring man. I felt so alone, even though we had four kids and the house was always rowdy and crowded. Sometimes I thought I'd go crazy with the frustration and anger and that's where the Valium helped. Now, I've started to emerge as a real person – and I have a lot of anger, which I think is healthy.'

By succumbing to the expectations and wishes of others, Anita was a prime candidate for depression. While she was only partly conscious of it, she was angry over her situation and feeling there was no alternative, she became depressed. Her Valium way of life was only part of the answer. Her anger was muted, but it was there all along. Valium took the edge off her anger and frustration. In hindsight, Anita recognises that she was lulled into a false sense of security. Jean Paul Sartre, the French existentialist philosopher, put it well when he said: *'We come to believe that these chains shall give us wings'.*

Lois Frankel is a therapist and author who links women's depression to women's anger. In her book, **Women, Anger and Depression**, she writes that anger is central to women's depression but often the woman cannot put a name to her 'brewing storm of emotions'. Dr. Frankel mentions that at one of her workshops, a woman told her, *'I feel at times that I will just implode'.*

It seems that loss, disappointment, anger and depression form a chainlink. Instead of aggression, the female response to disappointment or loss is depression. A research study in 1970 conducted by Dr. Alfred Friedman, found that depressed women are less verbally 'hostile' and 'aggressive' than non-depressed women. Dr. Friedman interpreted this tendency of the depressed woman to express very little verbal hostility in the following way:

> *'It may be that it is their (depressed women) inability to verbalise the hostility spontaneously to the person for whom they feel it at the time when it is appropriate (that) is part of their predisposition to become depressed. The tendency to deny the 'bad' in significant others and to perceive them selectively so they do not consciously become angry or depressed may be one of the ways to ward off a disturbed or depressive reaction.'*

These psychological theories dovetail with some of the views of the socialisation-of-women theory presented earlier. All these ideas are related to the sociological view that puts women, with their socialisation patterns and psychological tendencies, into the social context.

THE SOCIAL CONTEXT OF WOMEN'S LIVES

Brown and Harris are two English sociologists most readily identified with a sociological perspective on women's depression. In the mid-1970s they conducted a survey of approximately 500 women in an inner London suburb to examine the influence of social factors on the development of depression. They found that 15 per cent of the women were suffering from a 'definite affective (mood) disorder' and that 18 per cent were borderline cases. In other words, 33 per cent of the women interviewed were experiencing some degree of depression. Brown and Harris found that in 83 per cent of cases, traumatic life events or major ongoing difficulties in daily living preceded the onset of the women's depression.

The sociological view of women's depression then suggests that traumatic life events or ongoing difficulties trigger an experience of depression. These traumatic life events are called 'provoking agents' and usually involve a loss or disappointment concerning a person, object, role or idea. Bad relationships, unsatisfying work conditions and financial stresses are examples of ongoing difficulties.

It's thought that if a woman has such traumatic events and difficulties in her life and she has experienced what's called 'vulnerability factors', then her chances of having a depression are increased. These 'vulnerability factors' contribute to a woman's sense of low self-esteem, uncertainty and helplessness, making her vulnerable to the effects of loss and stress. There are four vulnerability factors:

- having three or more children under the age of 14 living at home
- lack of an intimate or confiding relationship
- loss of her mother in childhood
- lack of employment outside the home.

Putting together the psychological and sociological ideas gives a fuller picture of female vulnerability. This combined approach suggests that women have internalised society's prescriptions of 'feminine' behaviour and a stereotypically 'female' role can make a woman vulnerable to depression. Her vulnerability is likely to be increased by adverse social circumstances.

In my research and clinical experience, I've found that women are vulnerable to particular life stresses, strains and crisis points. Women are vulnerable to depression because of social expectations of who they should be. Women are vulnerable to depression because of society's expectations of how they should look. In an image-conscious society, only perfection will do for women. Women are vulnerable to depression because their relationships go wrong, break down and don't meet their needs. Women are vulnerable to depression during crisis points in their lives: during adolescence, in motherhood, at menopause. Women are vulnerable to depression when they're involved in the modern woman's juggling act: career-oriented yet having to do more than her fair share of the home duties.

While current social trends tend to allow women greater flexibility in behaviour and life-style, there is always a price to be paid. It seems that in the new millennium, being a woman is still a hazardous business.

3
IMAGES OF WOMEN

If it's a woman, it's caustic;
If it's a man, it's authoritative.

BARBARA WALTERS

Studies have shown that girls as young as four are more sociable and empathic while boys are less sociable, empathic and cooperative. What appears to happen is that boys in developing their masculine personality, are expected to deny their 'feminine' side, including strong relational and interdependent qualities. Girls, on the other hand, seem to relinquish their capacity for independence in response to love and approval. In essence, boys are bribed with a promise of power and domination, girls are rewarded for being nurturing and loving.

Parents have been observed to ask their 18 month-old girls how they are feeling more than they ask boys of the same age. Mothers also were found to talk to their two year old daughters about feelings more than they do to two year old sons.

As the young girl develops, she has a tendency to define herself in relation to others. As a woman, she is expected, more than a man, to be nurturant, to suppress anger and to be relatively nonassertive. It is interesting – and concerning – to note that these are the exact attributes that research has revealed as vulnerability factors relative to depression.

Today's society still views the female role with ambiguity. Expectations are often conflicting. A woman may be expected to fulfil two disparate roles – such as femme fatale and mother. A woman may be expected to conform to a very narrow and sometimes false image of femininity. Often, today's woman is expected to be all things to all people, inside the family and in the workplace.

Some women become depressed when they believe they fail to conform to expected roles and fit certain images. Because women are still presented with a rather narrow range of images with which to identify, there is the potential for women to feel they don't measure up. The gap between the ideal and their reality leaves them feeling depressed, with low self-esteem and a sense of defeatism.

It is true that women are no longer powerless. The women's liberation movement saw to that. In reality, women can say 'no' or 'yes' – though that doesn't mean they will. There is still a lot of pressure on a woman to be accommodating and nurturing.

WOMAN AS FEMME FATALE

It has been said that to be a woman is to be a femme fatale – a sex object. A woman is expected to be sexual in order to attract a man. But, once having attracted him, a woman is not then supposed to be too sexual, if she is to be seen as a 'nice girl'.

These contradictory messages make for some interesting tension. Just think of all the feelings of guilt and self-recrimination women could throw away if they refuse to take too much notice of these messages. As Anita Brookner points out in her novel, **Hotel du Lac**, *'Good women always think it is their fault when someone else is being offensive. Bad women never take the blame for anything'.*

Of course, a woman can enjoy being found attractive and feeling attractive. However, she can only enjoy these feelings if she is in a position to have some control. Many women report feeling a sense of emptiness, a nothingness which is part of their experience of depression. Liane, 42, comments,

> *'I was in a relationship for 15 years where I gave my husband everything he wanted without feeling anything much myself. I remember feeling numb and empty. I had sexual feelings, but they seemed to disappear whenever we had sex. I was always much more aware of his needs than my own. As for him, he didn't have a clue about my needs. Nor did he care. I remember when I called*

it quits, he was surprised. Everything had been fine for him. Typical, I thought. I've now met a wonderful man, who brings me alive sexually and my depression has lifted.'

Liane, like many women, felt she needed to subordinate her needs to those of her husband. What this meant was that she had 15 years of dissatisfaction and depression.

Some women don't see themselves this way. For them, their sexuality is much more confident and overt. More and more, women are being given permission to free themselves and feel better about themselves as sexual beings. Becoming assertive about your needs is important if you don't want to end up feeling depressed about yourself and your sexuality.

Claudia, 33, is married and works part-time as a sales assistant. She says she was always a 'good girl' until she read in a magazine about a female director who was making soft-porn videos for couples. Claudia had what her doctor called a 'low-grade depression' most of her married life. That magazine article helped Claudia understand that at least some of her depression was related to feeling sexually unsatisfied. She and her husband bought some of these videos, which were made from a woman's point of view, and watched them together. Claudia comments,

'These videos were very liberating for me. They are well made and not as silly as the ones that are usually made. They were erotic and sensual – but still a turn-on for my husband. We started experimenting more and discovered my real sexual side – I'd been hiding it from myself all those years. I started to feel good about myself as a woman and I started being more demanding sexually. I wasn't afraid anymore – I had needs and they were going to be met.'

But, in order to take control of her sexuality, a woman must be assertive. Or learn to be assertive. In the 1980s assertiveness became a buzz word for women. Yet, many women remain unassertive – about their needs, wants and views.

ASSERTIVE SKILLS

Research has found that assertive skills are learnt. Many women don't receive adequate training in these skills in their childhood. For instance, if as a child you are discouraged from expressing your opinions, this can lead to difficulties in later life when such skills are required. Your communication and conflict resolution skills may need to be developed.

Being assertive means that you behave in a way that demonstrates that you see yourself as equal to others. You do not see yourself as superior, which can be perceived as aggressive. And you do not see yourself as inferior, which can be seen by others as unassertive. Generally speaking, assertive behaviour is rational and reasonable, and demonstrates that you value yourself and others.

ASSERTIVENESS IS AN ISSUE FOR WOMEN

Stress and tension are caused by not expressing feelings directly. Your anger builds up when you replay situations in your mind. It becomes difficult for you to relax and you start having trouble sleeping.

Depression results from your negative feelings about contending with something you feel is wrong. Your unexpressed feelings start to haunt you. By avoiding speaking up, you start to feel helpless and powerless which also make you feel down.

Unassertive behaviour and aggressive behaviour result in loss of self-confidence and feeling down. They can also lead to loss of control. Unassertive behaviour causes loss of control of the situation and aggressive behaviour leads to loss of self-control.

CIRCLE THIS

Assertiveness is the ability to express your thoughts and feelings openly. It is the ability to stand up for your rights. Assertiveness is an important skill for a number of reasons:

- it can help you develop close, warm relationships
- it can give you the means of getting positive responses from others
- it allows other people to understand you better

We are told that the modern woman is liberated. Yet, some women are being constrained by unrealistic and outdated images. Another image of women which can lead to depression is that of the ideal mother.

WOMAN AS MOTHER

On the flip side of the coin to the young, sexy, desirable slim woman image is that of the sexless maternal being whose sole role in life is to serve men and children. These images are depicted in advertising, in movies and television, and reinforced by the Madonna/Whore distinction many people carry around in their heads. Maureen is 48 and has only ever known life from the point of view of the traditional homemaker role. Her children have left home and Maureen has been depressed since. She says:

'My doctor tells me I have a serious case of 'empty-nest syndrome'. All my life, I was someone's wife and mother – that's how I saw myself – that was my job. Now, there's only my husband and me left at home – things seem dismal.

'I guess over the years we grew apart without knowing it and now that the kids are gone we don't have much in common. Life is not very meaningful anymore. It's funny, but when I was younger and busy with the kids and the house I wasn't half as exhausted as I am now – everything seems to overwhelm me.

'Lately I've taken to ignoring the housework – I feel useless and unmotivated. I don't have half the responsibilities I used to have, but what I do have I've abandoned. Just before my husband insisted I see a doctor, I'd spent about a week in bed. I remember thinking, why get up? So I just stayed in bed.'

In Maureen's case, the loss of the traditional homemaker role with its well-defined expectations and rewards, was enough to trigger her depression. Many women find security in the homemaker role and a tremendous sense of satisfaction. When the rewards of motherhood are no longer there, these women feel lost and lonely. Very often the rift in their relationship with their husbands has gone unnoticed until only the two of them are left in the house. Then, a situation which has always been, becomes magnified and sometimes the couple find that only separation or divorce heals their pain.

For other women, like Barbara, 54, the homemaker role was experienced as too constraining and oppressive. Her chronic depression lifted when her maternal responsibilities lightened and her children left home. She comments:

'I always found the chaos of home life with four kids maddening. There was always too much noise, too many meals to prepare, too many rooms to clean and too much ferrying of children around all weekend.

'My husband had a high-powered job so I was pretty well on my own. We were in a position to get some help in at times – but really the buck stopped with me. I was the mother. I was supposed to be all things to all people. I married young and for thirty-two years, I as a person, was driven underground.

'When my last child left home I celebrated. Some of my friends thought I was crazy – other people passed judgement on me as a heartless mother, how could I and all that – I thought I had every right to celebrate my rebirth. For thirty-two years, I felt stretched to the limit and I used to get terribly depressed about it all – but I had to carry on.

'I had to submerge myself for the good of the family. I'm now my own person and loving it. I love my husband and my children, but I'm not their servant or saviour anymore. I've never felt happier. I'm doing an art course and dabbling with some painting. Every morning I get up looking forward to a day as a person, instead of as a mother.'

The messages that women receive about their roles are strong, unrelenting and delivered almost daily. From a young age, girls are taught that to be valued they must conform. Conforming to the sexy image, the maternal image and the 'good girl' image are necessary if the woman wants acceptance.

WOMAN AS FEMININE – BE A GOOD GIRL

'Little girls should...' is a line girls often hear. This 'should' system of operating in the world may lead to depression. For many girls and women, 'shoulds' become the masters of their destiny. The biggest 'should' perhaps is the idea that to be feminine is to be nice all the time. Women are not supposed to get angry.

Think about it. All the images of angry women are derogatory – the witch, the bitch, the shrew and the vixen. On the other hand, an angry man is considered to be showing admirable strength. Barbara Walters in the quote at the beginning of this chapter highlights this difference in perception: *'If it's a woman, it's caustic; If it's a man, it's authoritative'.*

One theory suggests that depression results from a suppression of aggressive feelings. Instead of being angry with others, the woman might turn her anger on herself. This leads to an attack on her sense of worth and integrity and she gets depressed.

Some studies suggest that when a woman deviates from her expected feminine sex-role, society and even mental health professionals may question her so-called 'femininity'. They may even question her mental health. It's no wonder that women, subject as they are to certain role expectations are vulnerable to anxiety and depression.

English psychiatrist Jane Price, says that:

'Women still find it difficult to express anger and when they do express it in ways which society would consider appropriate for men, they are usually condemned as mad, bad or unwomanly.'

Kathy Nairne and Gerrilyn Smith, two English feminist psychologists believe that the most damaging aspect of the idea of femininity is the pressure to be nice all the time. Repressing anger in order to preserve your sense of female identity they say, *'can lead to an attack on our own sense of worth and so to depression'.*

The messages around anger are clear and strong. They are linked to a woman's sense of self and femininity. Women learn to repress their angry feelings at an early age. It's not only men who give women the message that anger is unacceptable. A girl's mother may influence her regarding what is acceptable or not. Mothers impart ideas and values and often these are consistent with stereotyped behaviour for boys and girls.

Sara was the only girl in her family. She is a 22 year old student who is beginning to come to terms with her repressed anger and obvious depression. She says:

'When we were growing up, mom would encourage my brothers to stand up for themselves, to be angry, aggressive and perhaps even to get physical if they

> were being bullied or dealt with unfairly. On the other hand, I was told to 'turn the other cheek' and be 'ladylike' and not show my anger. While my brothers were told to defend themselves, I was told to remember `Sticks and stones will break my bones, but words will never hurt me'. What a joke! Words are very hurtful, but I had to hide my anger. It just wasn't fair.'

To be feminine is to be passive. To be passive is not to take initiative. It means not acting for yourself. Consequently, girls grow up believing that the main fulfilment in life will come in the form of a relationship. A relationship validates their worth. Many women still wait to be chosen by a man.

While the perennial 'bad boy' receives 'should' messages that reinforce his strength and initiative, little girls are encouraged to be clean, cautious and tidy. They must wait for life to happen. Girls are not encouraged to be adventurous. Boys, on the other hand, are encouraged to be explorers and warriors.

Denella, 27, is a nurse and recognises how her depression was related to being bombarded with messages as a child about how she should be. She says:

> 'As a teenager I was very rebellious – and angry. Only I think I was a rebel with a cause. My parents were always telling me I should be this way or that way – but never as I was. I would do outrageous things to get them stirred up – and I guess I was different. But it took me a long time to celebrate my difference. Although I was acting up and doing things I shouldn't have I wasn't all that sure of myself. I was depressed really – because I was different and being told I shouldn't be. It didn't stop me from rebelling, but I had lots of private doubts and I coped with my depression by getting it out in music and song.'

Part of Denella's problem was she wasn't concerned with clothes and make-up. Her mother, in particular, thought Denella 'should' have been. Of course, concern with our appearance can be seen as a form of self-expression, a form of play. It can be seen as a means of pleasure. But, if women feel pressurised by the images of female beauty then their failure to live up to the images can well lead to depression.

Fashions change often, even to the extent of whether women should have large or small breasts. Recently, one prominent women's magazine sported a cover headline: 'Small breasts are back'. Where does that fashion trend leave the large-breasted woman? And what of the small-breasted woman, who for so many years, was made to feel inadequate? In reality, breasts are breasts and they come in all shapes and sizes. However, women have become accustomed to having their bodies defined in fashion cycle terms.

Sally is a 25 year old physical therapist who has struggled with the 'feminine' dilemma for years. She comments:

> *'Although it makes me very depressed, I think I've bought into the whole image of the female and the female body. What is acceptable and how I should strive for perfection as a woman. I sometimes wonder why I dress the way I do. Is it for me? Or am I trying to be feminine and attract men? I'm deeply affected by this dilemma – because it seems so superficial – but deep at the same time. I mean, why don't I feel feminine without presenting myself in a particular way?'*

Women are judged more on their looks than are men. Women are expected to be fatless, spotless and hairless. The ultimate irony is that the 'real' woman, the 'feminine' woman is to wear make-up and change her appearance in such a way as to become unlike her 'real' self – she must conform to a 'false' but 'feminine' image of herself.

Women also are expected to be emotional. How many times have you heard the adage, 'men are rational and women are emotional'? This means that women are permitted, perhaps even expected to cry easily, while such behaviour is taboo in a man.

WOMEN WEEP, MEN DON'T

One theory holds that women cry because it's safer than becoming angry. Simone de Beauvoir wrote, *'Women's aptitude for facile (easy) tears comes largely from the fact that her life is built upon a foundation of impotent revolt'*.

Since the physician Hippocrates claimed that hysteria was caused by a wandering uterus, a tendency to weep has been closely identified with women. Tearfulness and helplessness are regarded as 'feminine' ways of being. Such emotional expression is almost expected in women. When women don't show emotion, they are said to be 'cold', 'uncaring' 'icy' or worse.

Women are emotional and 'neurotic'. Very rarely is a man labelled 'neurotic'. But the expectation that a woman is weak, submissive and in need of guidance lest she lose her way in the world is part of the myth about women being highly emotional human beings.

In the 1950s and 1960s, social scientists told us that men are 'instrumental' and 'task-oriented' and women are 'expressive' and 'person-oriented'. Put simply, they were saying that men are rational and cool-headed and need to be so to survive in the workplace. Women, on the other hand, are emotional and nurturing, because this best suits them to motherhood.

Many of these sex stereotypes have been challenged in recent years, yet people still hold firm views about the truth of these stereotypes. That such ideas endure is no surprise. Small children get clear messages early in life – feminine and masculine behaviour emerges with encouragement.

Researchers have sat behind one-way screens and watched the behaviour of women towards girl and boy babies. When the women were told that the baby was a girl, they behaved as if it was and rocked the child and spoke quietly to it. They were also vigilant about not letting the child explore too much. However, when the women were told that the baby was a boy, they again behaved as if it was and were much more encouraging of the child's play and spoke more loudly to it. What is interesting is that at times the women were duped into believing that a girl child was a boy and vice versa – and they behaved according to the false information they were given. In this way, girls and boys are 'schooled' to varying degrees to be what girls and boys should be. The expectations are clear.

This means that women and men occupy different places in the social landscape of life. They are expected to do so. Almost from birth we are steered towards different expectations of us. Female and male behaviour is, in part, dictated by such expectations.

Men may drink and be thought to be masculine, but women are said to show emotion. One doctor whom I interviewed said, *'I have a theory* that under similar stresses and strains, women get depressed and men turn to alcohol'.

This view is confirmed by Annette. She is a 48 year old married woman who works as a lawyer. She says:

'I've noticed a difference between my husband and me. When I get down and depressed, I have what I call the 'weeps'. I just cry and cry. This happened when my mother died. All I can remember doing for weeks was crying. My loss was so great. Even at work, I'd occasionally burst into tears during the day.

'But when my husband's father died, he appeared very stoic. I was surprised he didn't shed a tear – I was very judgemental at the time – accusing him of being heartless. He responded by saying something like 'women cry to release their emotions, men usually don't'. I was puzzled, because he'd been so close to his father – he respected him so. What I did notice was that he started drinking more at night. Not enough to be labelled alcoholic or anything – he'd always had a few drinks after work, but after his father died, he had about six drinks every night for about five months. I guess it was his way of dealing with his emotions. It's an interesting difference. I've spoken to friends about it and some of them have noticed the same thing. It's the difference between men and women.'

Annette articulates a point of view which reinforces yet again, the effects of socialisation on women – and men. It is acceptable for women to weep, but for a man to show such blatant emotion might call attention to his 'feminine' side. Such attention generally is considered undesirable and very early in life, boys are conditioned to be 'tough' and often they are physically disciplined if they show emotions – a sure sign of weakness. What Annette calls 'the difference between men and women', appears to be alive and well in our world, as we struggle with issues of equality between the sexes.

If Simone de Beauvoir is right, women should learn to become appropriately assertive.

SWINGING BETWEEN BEING UNASSERTIVE AND AGGRESSIVE

Do you recognise the pattern? You are irritated by something but you do not act directly to resolve it. Gradually, your irritation grows and you feel like a walking time bomb. One day, a small annoyance sets you off. It goes something like this. Those bottled up feelings cause an explosion. And you feel like you've lost control. You feel anxious, demoralised, guilty and low. You may be concerned that you will lose control again, so in future similarly irritating situations, you don't speak up. The cycle can repeat itself endlessly. It's up to you to break the cycle.

HOW TO FEEL MORE IN CONTROL

By being assertive, you will feel more in control of situations. This in turn reduces stress and depression. Research into depression suggests that assertive behaviour can help to prevent further experiences of the blues.

Assertive behaviour means treating yourself well. It means doing the best you can to make sure others will respect you and treat you this way. Assertive behaviour leads to mutual respect.

BECOMING AN ASSERTIVE WOMAN

STEP ONE – RECOGNISE YOUR UNASSERTIVE BEHAVIOURS

Unassertive behaviours leave you feeling powerless and low. Unassertive women have difficulty expressing their thoughts, feelings and wishes directly.

Learn to be direct. Ask for what you want, within reason. Confront problems and attempt to resolve them before they get out of hand. Don't suffer by fence-sitting when you can make it known what you want. Take control.

STEP TWO – USE YOUR PERSONAL ASSERTIVE RIGHTS

There are personal assertive rights which are available to everyone. If you are not allowing yourself these rights then you are denying yourself the benefit of being assertive. Read through the following list and note how many of these rights you are using. Begin using ones that are new for you.

Bill of Assertive Rights

- I have the right to be treated as a competent person
- I have the right to my own values; others have a right to their values
- I have the right to feel and express my feelings, including anger; others have the right to express their feelings
- I have the right not to be labelled, but to be treated as an individual
- I have the right to make mistakes and be responsible for them; others have the right to make mistakes and accept the consequences
- I have the right to change my mind; others have the right to change their minds
- I have the right to make my own decisions; others have the same right
- I have the right to refuse requests without feeling guilty or making excuses
- I have the right to recognise my needs are as important as others' needs
- I have the right to ask for affection, help, support; other people have the right to ask for these things

Exercise — Learning to use your personal rights

If after reading the Bill of Assertive Rights you find you're not using all your personal rights, nominate ones to work on as weekly or monthly goals. You may find it useful to pin up this bill of rights somewhere in your home as a reminder of what you are entitled to as an assertive woman.

STEP 3 – TALK YOURSELF INTO ASSERTION

Your thinking can block assertive behaviour. Look at some of the following examples:

- Assuming that you know how others will react:
  - *'She'll be upset if I say...'*
  - *'He'll think I'm stupid if...'*

- Putting negative labels on assertive behaviour:
  - *'I don't want to seem rude...'*

- 'It's bad manners to...'
- Talking yourself out of how you feel or rationalising:
  - 'Oh, it's not that bad...'
  - 'She's only saying that for my own good...'
- Talking yourself out of the responsibility for assertive action:
  - 'I can't change things anyway...'
  - 'It'll all work out...'
- Believing your strong feelings are right and others are wrong or believing feelings are facts:
  - 'I feel put down, therefore I was'
  - 'I feel he hates me...'
- Taking too much responsibility for another person's feelings, and blaming yourself if someone gets angry or hurt as a result of you being assertive. Remember, if you have been reasonable, rational and non-aggressive, it is not your fault that someone feels the way they do. They may be overreacting. You have no control over how another person thinks. You are doing yourself a disservice if you allow other people's reactions to stop you from being assertive
- Setting limits and restrictions on when to be assertive:
  - 'The other person must be able to handle it'
  - 'I'll say it if the time is right'

Be kind to yourself. Remind yourself that you matter and that your feelings are as important as those of other people. You have rights, and others have rights. Recognise that feelings are not right or wrong, they just exist. You have the right to let others know your thoughts and feelings and ask that they be respected. Other people have similar rights, which you should respect.

(Steps 1,2 and 3: Adapted from Tanner and Ball, 1989)

> **CIRCLE THIS**

Remind yourself of your bill of rights. Memorise each of the rights. Give yourself as many rights as you give others. Treat yourself as well as you treat others. Practise telling yourself your rights – stand up for yourself and don't feel exploited.

BUILDING YOUR SKILLS BY SETTING ASSERTIVENESS TASKS

You can build your repertoire of skills by deciding on daily, weekly and monthly exercises in assertion. Choose easy situations at first. Practice your assertiveness and build up to more difficult situations.

Rehearse and plan what you want to say and do. It may be useful to write it out if you feel anxiety will make you go blank in the actual situation.

> **CIRCLE THIS**

Being assertive takes practice. And practice and practice. All skills require practice. Be consistent and persistent, and then even more consistent and persistent! Don't just try once and give up. Be firm and stick to your plan to develop your assertiveness skills. Resolve to keep trying new assertiveness skills and improving on them.

The key to success is perseverance and practice.

WOMEN AND 'THE FEMININE MYSTIQUE'

Betty Friedan calls it 'the problem that has no name'. It is a problem which exists today, but in a diluted form. When Betty Friedan was making her observations and calling public attention to the problem without a name, women had elaborate hair-styles, constraining clothes and took the advice of Dr. Spock. At that time, women said they didn't want careers. They were told they shouldn't have careers. Guilt was reinforced by the prevailing theories of maternal deprivation. It was an era when women's dissatisfaction and depression was interpreted as a personal failure. What Friedan saw as the 'quiet desperation' of anger and despair and called 'the problem with no name', was dubbed by a doctor as 'the housewife's syndrome'.

Ironically, many women in the 1950s and 1960s did not lack things. Materially, they had too much. However, they felt that their lives were empty. Many were depressed – caught between not knowing who they were or what they wanted to become. Betty Friedan wrote:

> *"The problem lay buried, unspoken for many years in the minds of American women. It was a strong stirring, a sense of dissatisfaction, a yearning that women suffered in the middle of the twentieth century in the United States. Each suburban wife struggled with it alone. As she made the beds, shopped for groceries, matched slip cover material, ate peanut butter sandwiches, chauffeured Cub Scouts and Brownies, lay beside her husband at night, she was afraid to ask even of herself the silent question: 'Is this all?'"*

Images of women have remained static, yet changed in the years since Friedan raised our consciousness. 'Is this all?' might well be on the lips of today's woman. It's a case of the old adage, 'The more things change, the more they remain the same'.

Remember this: Betty Friedan also said, *'In the end, a woman, as a man, has the power to choose and to make her own heaven or hell'.*

DEVELOPING A BETTER ATTITUDE TOWARDS YOURSELF

Attitudes towards yourself can affect your mood. Maybe you've taken on board attitudes that are not positive to your self-esteem. If you want to hook into the positive or upward spiral, then you have to be aware how you perceive yourself and how you behave. Are you inhibited by low self-esteem and self-confidence? If you are, then it's time to examine how you can improve your self-esteem and gain more confidence.

Although self-esteem and self-confidence are often used as if they were one and the same thing, they do have different meanings.

Self-esteem refers to how you judge yourself. What are the personal values, beliefs and attitudes which affect how you react in situations? Examples of positive beliefs and assumptions which enhance self-esteem are:

- *'I know I'm a worthwhile person and I can accept criticism.'*
- *'Everyone is human. It is okay to have limitations in what I can do.'*

- *'We all make mistakes. I can accept my mistakes and retain self-respect.'*

Self-confidence comes from the specific things that you do. For instance, you can build up confidence when you gain a sense of achievement or satisfaction from attempting challenging tasks. You may not feel confident the first time you play tennis, but as you practise, your confidence will build. When you've got the blues, your self-confidence gets tested. You undergo a set-back and you feel less confident about performing as well as you would like.

DID YOU KNOW THAT SOME BELIEFS CAN UNDERMINE YOUR SELF-ESTEEM?

Some beliefs held by women make them vulnerable to the blues. For instance, believing that you must have everyone's approval all of the time and that you are only worthwhile through your achievements can lead to a sense of vulnerability. Similarly, women who hold the view that they must do things perfectly or not at all and have unrealistic expectations that the world be a fair and just place, can have their self-esteem eroded and feel vulnerable to depression.

YOU CAN IMPROVE YOUR SELF-ESTEEM BY...

Being yourself
Stop trying to prove yourself. You are as worthwhile as anyone else. By trying to satisfy an unrealistic belief like 'I must be the perfect woman', you are missing out on the important things in life. Accept yourself for who you are. Be yourself. Love yourself, warts and all!

Knowing your positive points
Modesty is not a virtue, particularly if it makes you feel low and vulnerable. You need to be able to recognise your skills and achievements. You need to feel good about them.

Develop the habit of reflecting on positive statements you can make about yourself. Get to know your positive points when you feel good about yourself, write them down and then read them to yourself when you feel down. For ready reference, keep a copy close to hand.

Exercise: Create positive thoughts about yourself

Now it's time to put your plan into action. Reflect on your positive qualities. Write them down, or tape them – and read or listen to all those good qualities that make up you.

Be definite when you create positive thoughts about yourself. Don't say vague things like, 'I suppose I'm kind and caring', say 'I know I'm a compassionate person'. Rather than saying, 'I guess I've got a sense of humor', say 'I know that I can be bright and witty'. Rather than saying, 'I guess I can do my job', say, 'I enjoy my work and I know I am competent'.

Some sample positive thoughts

- I'm generous with my friends
- I know I look good when I make an effort and get dressed up
- I know that some people find me good company
- I will try to keep working on myself and developing new skills
- It's okay to be lazy/angry at times, because that's part of being human
- I am competent, but I don't have to be perfect

RESPECTING YOURSELF

Learn to treat yourself well. If you respect yourself, then others will too. Don't put yourself down – and never in front of others. Challenge others who put you down. Allow yourself the experience of pleasant activities and give yourself rewards. Praise yourself if you've completed a task. Treat yourself as you would a very good friend. Be kind to yourself. Becoming a self-respecting person will keep you away from that downward spiral into the blues.

And now, for a daily exercise all women should do to keep the blues at bay. At first you might think it's too tall an order to ask that you think of five positive thoughts about yourself – but with practice you'll find you can do it easily! If you can think of more than five – don't stop there! Take your time in doing this exercise. Reflect, and write in as much detail as you can. In the beginning, you may feel self-conscious, but remember, this list is your private list – so don't be shy, and help yourself by being positive!

> **Exercise** **Five positive thoughts**
>
> At the end of each day, write a list of five positive thoughts about yourself and your experiences. Keep this list and add to it daily.

By concentrating on your good points, what you do well, how good you look, instead of dwelling on the negative, you will feel better about yourself.

CIRCLE THIS

Remember, it's up to you – as Betty Friedan says, you have 'the power to choose'. Develop strong self-esteem, feel positively about yourself – and overturn that blue feeling!

Another image that creates a sense of depression for many women has to do with their body. Body image can become an obsession for some women. Many of these women have poor self-esteem, become depressed and believe they are not good enough. For many women with perfectly normal and attractive bodies, their constant striving for an unrealistic ideal leads to a sense of depression. They develop a distorted view of their bodies – not seeing themselves as they are. Often eating disorders and depression go hand-in-hand.

WOMEN AND BODY IMAGE IMAGES

Deirdre is telling me how low she feels. She has the sort of 'glamour' job many women envy. She is 33 and has been a fashion buyer for a major retail store for five years. She travels, she wines, she dines and she meets interesting people. But she's now a size 14. Ten years ago, she was a size 10. She says to me,

> *'I don't feel like a proper woman anymore. I don't feel desirable. I was so happy when I was a size 10, but look at me now – I look hideous – and in my line of business, image is everything. I've been dieting for about eight months but it's not making a big impact. About a year ago, I split up with my boyfriend. We'd been together six years and I'm sure he left because I was getting fat. I think about what happened a lot and I can't see any other good reason for him to quit the relationship.'*

The female body is in the public domain. Everyone it seems owns the female body. This means that the female body, over the past twenty years, has been shaped and sculpted to the 'ideal' image – the look of the supermodel.

It's no wonder that Deirdre feels like she's not a 'proper woman'. After all, she's two sizes from the ideal – and in what's considered the wrong direction. Of course, to Deirdre's mind, all her troubles are related to her body size. She even attributes her failed relationship to her increase in dress size. Socialisation clearly is at play here, together with some of that faulty thinking the cognitive psychologists talk about – Deirdre's view of herself, her world and her future is based on some fundamental false assumptions about happiness. But would Deirdre believe that? Probably not, because she's conditioned to feel good about herself only when she believes she's at her most lovable and valuable – a size 4.

Of course, it might be argued that the female body has always been in the public domain. Call it the tyranny of Venus, but in every age, the idealisation of the female form has taken on almost mystical proportions. In every age, the 'perfect body' takes one form only. The classical Greeks' notions of the perfect female body were about symmetry. They dictated that the distance between the nipples, the distance from the lower edge of the breast to navel and the distance from navel to the crotch be equal length – and that was the perfect body.

During the Renaissance, there was an emphasis on buxsomness, but by Victorian times, a lady was required to have an eighteen-inch waist. In the 1920's, the flat-chested flapper reigned supreme but by the mid-fifties, Marilyn Monroe's feminine beauty drew attention to curves – the hour-glass shape of breasts, nipped waists and hips.

Today's perfection is one of slimness. Breast size fashions come and go, but overall slimness stays. Slimness as femininity and femininity as slimness. Youth is associated with slimness. The 'Beautiful People' – are sculpted and pared down. How ordinary women see and experience their bodies is dictated by social and fashion forces outside of their control.

Deirdre is not alone in her body-image depression. A British couturier recently said: 'Very few women are happy with their bodies.'

Not long ago, a young female student of mine, Kara, already depressed about how 'big' she is, came to class visibly distressed. She had been given some unsolicited feedback by a group of road-side workers. She was angry about what she saw as their insensitivity and their assumption that they have the right to call her names as she minds her business and walks the public streets. This young, attractive woman of 21 has a big frame and can best be described as stocky. That's her genetic heritage. It's not her fault. She already feels guilty about not being 'thinner' – but the truth is, she can't be thinner. Nature did not mean her to be thin. She comments,

> 'I diet and diet, but I've got this big bone structure and even when I've dieted all the fat off my body, I look big. I don't know if I'll ever accept myself. It doesn't help when you're feeling so low about yourself and some scum decide to put the boot in. It's very demoralising.'

Kara is well-proportioned and has the sort of body which would have been appreciated in the 1950s. But she doesn't conform to today's ideal or perfect body. Not many of us do. However, many women do get depressed about their bodies. Insecurities breed depression.

EATING DISORDERS AND WOMEN

Food has always been symbolic as well as sustaining. In many ways, food as a symbol has never been more powerful than today. A primary school teacher recently revealed to me that she believes girls as young as nine are 'dieting' in order to remain 'slim'. Summer camps for overweight children offer the opportunity of having fun and losing weight at the same time. Nevertheless, it's easy to overlook the tremendous pressure on young women to conform to unnatural slimness.

Society's messages around food are contradictory and many women become hostages to these mixed messages. Zerbe writing in her book, *The Body Betrayed* says:

> 'Eating disorders are now recognised as major medical and psychiatric problems, affecting millions of women in the United States and Europe. Additionally of late we seem to be immersed in a symptomatic sea of

disordered eating among all women. Women's magazines tout the advantages of the latest fad diets side by side with pages of luscious recipes of America's nouvelle cuisine.'

On a simple level, food can be seen as a comfort for worry and anxiety and feelings of emptiness. Food can also be used to stuff down frustration, anger and depression which cannot be expressed. Still on another level, food can be denied because of what it represents – fullness and perhaps a sense of being out-of-control.

Food may represent an internalised split – good and bad. Good food represents a good person. Lettuce, low calorie, cold, bland, low fat food means becoming slim, successful, in control, lean, fit and sexy. Bad food such as high calorie, rich, thick, creamy, spicy and appetizing food means becoming a bad person – fat, out-of-control, unsuccessful, full, greedy and desiring.

If you are significantly overweight, it may help to think about what your weight means to you. Some women carry around excess pounds as a sheild against the world. A client, Caitlin, 34, told me that she would only admit to herself that her extra pounds were a protection. As far as the world was concerned, she was trying to lose weight – and occasionally she would lose a few pounds. When she did lose weight, she found people noticed, commented and congratulated her. But as Caitlin confided:

'The positive comments were not rewarding enough to overcome the deep need I felt to have that extra weight cushioning me from the world. My pounds were my protection – not that I would admit that outside the therapy room.'

Caitlin's need to have her pounds protect her, while at the same time, appear to want to shed this protection was conscious. For other women, this need is deeply embedded – and unconscious.

Depression often precedes eating disorders. It can also result from the inner turmoil and the dependence on control mechanisms to which some women become slaves. In a sense, food and the eating of it takes on a highly symbolic significance. The split between good and bad is reflected by society which subtley gives messages to women how much real control and choice they have about how they should be. While there seems to be more equality and opportunity for women today, there are also other powerful forces which constrain options and suggest images over which women have little control.

In one sense, women are in an ambivalent social position. They are told they can be high-achievers, go-getters, aggressive, 'out there' and even 'Superwoman'. However, in another sense, women must remain 'pretty', 'cute', 'passive' and slim to be valued. While women are told it's acceptable to be independent and strong, their presentation of self – their appearance is still a key way in which they are judged. Many TV anchorwomen disappear after the age of 35 and the more successful ones are referred to as 'women of a certain age' in tones of wonderment that they should still command huge audiences and high salaries.

Some women grow up with a sense that they are 'good' when they are controlled and 'in control' and 'bad' when they are not in control. Such women have little concept of themselves as people with rights and sensibilities – they see themselves as objects.

Such a woman might say, 'I hate the trap my body puts me in – I hate my body and the way I feel about myself. I only feel good when I don't eat.'

THE PROBLEM OF BODY IMAGE

Dr Alexander Lowen in his book ***The Betrayal of the Body***, said, *'A healthy person has an image of herself that agrees with the way her body looks and feels'.* With so much pressure around today to look and feel differently from the way women do, it's no wonder there's a lot of unhappiness and body-image depression. In her book, ***Body Traps***, Dr Judith Roden refers to diet-induced depression among women. Oprah Winfrey, 'the Queen of the talk-shows', has been quoted as saying that she considered losing weight and a newly acquired svelte body as her biggest achievement. Considering all her achievements, it's a big statement to make.

Women in their teens, twenties, thirties and beyond may be harbouring an image of themselves as fat, ugly, awkward and unfeminine, because they are themselves and not the rangy cat-walk models featured in magazines. Often women become depressed because they are fixated on one particular 'fault' or 'flaw' in their appearance. Their breasts are too small, too large, their tummies are not flat enough, their pecs are not tight enough, their arms are too hairy, their hips too fat, their nose too prominent and their chin too weak. With the help of plastic surgery these fatal flaws can now be 'corrected'.

Statistics tell us that in the United States, the plastic or cosmetic surgery industry is a $300 million a year business. Every year, thousands of women go under the surgeon's scalpel to cut away their unhappiness with their appearance. There is more and more pressure on women to dislike what they see in the mirror.

Women read about the marvels of cosmetic surgery in the glossy women's magazines. They jealously pore over the 'before-and-after' photos of those women who've been 'made-over' surgically. The message they are being given is simple: Looking better will magically translate into a happier and more satisfying life.

This message is irrational. But when a women is feeling vulnerable and low, she's not in a state to do any reality-testing. In fact, she's at her most vulnerable to suggestive, seductive advertising about cosmetic surgery. Maybe the woman is ready to receive the message of dramatic before-and-after photos which boast the headline: 'She's Found New Confidence'.

Cosmetic surgery advertisements play on women's insecurities. Many cosmetic surgeons market themselves – and their services – aggressively. In one advertisement, a statuesque blonde is clad in revealing red leather, exhibiting an uplift most women only dream about, and the text tells us that she is dressed by North Beach Leather and 'Surgical Sculpture by Franklin A. Rose, MD'.

In Houston, Texas, where the first breast augmentation took place in 1962, breasts are ubiquitous. The *Texas Monthly* magazine recently dubbed Houston, 'silicone city' and said:

> *'Plastic surgery ads featuring young women with bountiful bosoms figure prominently in local health and fitness magazines ('Summer's here. Time to look your best')... a shift from an oil-based to a breast-based economy... Houston's relationship with the breast makes for a modern morality tale, one that says a lot about the fantasies and ambitions of a city, and how those dreams have changed the way women look around the world.'*

Projections reveal that over 100,000 American women will have breast implant surgery in any year. Who can blame the woman who is depressed and insecure, low in self-esteem, for falling prey to such powerful messages. A few years ago, I read that at a Paris fashion show, tailoring of clothing had been surpassed by tailoring of the body – by cosmetic procedure. A cat-walk model disappears behind a screen, has a little injection and comes out with generous, sensuous lips. It's simply that easy. That's the message.

The comedian Joan Rivers has quipped: *'Looks count. Forget 'inner beauty'. If a man wants inner beauty, he'll take X-rays.'* Such comments reinforce the social pressures on women to consult surgeons to redeal the hand that nature dealt them. Forget genetics, forget time, the cosmetic surgeon has the panacea.

Back in 1968, a study by psychiatrists revealed that women expressed greater dissatisfaction with their bodily parts than men. Since that time, this sense of dissatisfaction has snowballed, as the media and women's magazines display images of the ideal woman relentlessly. We have a daily diet of how we should look and mostly, we don't measure up.

It seems that 'up' is the way many women request their breast size. Surgeons describe how a decade ago women typically were requesting a B cup. Today, the request is for a C and increasingly a D cup. As one wit quipped, *'Are we talking breast sizes or levels of the women's self-esteem here?'*

But can women who are depressed because of their apparent deficits in the body department be blamed for buying the message? It's a powerful message we're given every day: To be female means to be perfect. Women, unlike men, are not prized for 'quirky' looks. One woman who has bought the message about physical perfection is Lisa.

Lisa, 37, is an attractive blonde who dresses impeccably. She is a legal secretary and a plastic surgery junkie. At 22, she had a nose job, at 28, she had breast implants and at 33, she had liposuction of the stomach and thighs. All these procedures were undertaken by her to be more attractive, feel better about herself and in her general pursuit of happiness. The only problem is that she tells me she's more depressed about her body image than she's ever been.

She says:

'I thought if I had all this work done on me I'd be a happier person. I thought I'd be a better person and I'd be admired and I'd have to beat off the guys. Only it hasn't happened that way. I keep thinking that if I had more work done on me then I'd be better. It's a bit of a vicious cycle.

"I recently read about some woman who's got Barbie doll as her role model and she's had 45 operations. Even I think that's going over the top. And I think she's an airhead saying that Barbie is her ideal woman. But I also think that maybe I should have cheek and chin implants to balance my face more and then maybe when I'm 40, I'll have a face-lift.

'I know it doesn't make any sense. I say I've had plastic surgery and it hasn't changed my life, but then I keep thinking, maybe I'd be less depressed if I had one more thing done – maybe I'd be better and happier.'

Maybe – and then maybe not. Julaine, 23, works as a hair-stylist and has always been what she calls 'image-conscious'. She dresses in a trendy, slightly wacky way – always at the cutting edge of fashion. She says:

'I've always been into hair, clothes, make-up – you know, wanting to look my best. Like I'm not a raving beauty really, but I do my best. I work in an industry where it's all image, image, image. It's like everyone's competing – all the time. I used to get real depressed because my boobs were small. I'm not a big person, but I was flat as a pancake.

'So I saved up and bought new boobs. I was real pleased with them at first. I used to show them off all the time. But then my boobs began to hurt and they felt like they were turning to stone. I had to have them redone. And this time, they've been in for over a year and they're fine. But I'm still depressed about my appearance. It's like I won't be happy until I'm perfect. Funny isn't it? Well, not real funny, but you know what I mean. I'm going to have my nose straightened out as soon as I've saved up enough money. I know I'll feel better about myself then.'

Again, maybe and maybe not. Maybe Julaine will never be happy with herself.

Unfortunately for some women, their body-image is a source of depression for much of their lives. We all know women who've dieted for years, purged for decades and still not found their way out of the maze. They remain depressed. Their self-esteem is low. They are trapped in the mind-set that to be slim is to be beautiful and nothing else will do.

One woman who has worked through her body-image depression and come out on the other side is Beverley, 46. Beverley owns a delightful gift shop and has the sort of personality which attracts people to her. She says she struggled with her weight for three decades and finally found she'd developed enough self-esteem and confidence to 'give up the struggle'. She worries about her two teenage daughters and their attitudes to food and dieting. She says:

> 'I believe it all started with the Duchess of Windsor. You know, 'no woman can be too thin or too rich' – well, she was both! This fear of fat, of being overweight has reached epidemic proportions among women today. I bought into it for about thirty years. I felt that if I was slim, I was good and I would be more valued. But my natural body shape is on the curvaceous side so it was a real struggle for me. But over the years, I'd had a number of successes in business and I got a lot of kudos – and I'm in a very supportive relationship. My husband loves me for who I am – that's given me a tremendous amount of confidence. Ten pounds either way doesn't make any difference to him. I'm still me.
>
> 'But I worry about my daughters. They're both at a vulnerable age and I fear for them – and their sanity. You know, it's hard for teenage girls to listen to their mum – I try, but I think all my good advice falls on deaf ears.'

A FINAL WORD ABOUT IMAGES

Images encourage women to live up to ideals which are unrealistic and mostly, unrealisable. There's a social message which women receive that those who don't live up to such images are failures. Failing to meet such ideals can be a depressing experience.

Many women live with long-term feelings of low self-esteem, self-doubt and self-deprecation because they don't or can't conform to the ideal.

It seems there will always be images of women which are contradictory. When an image attempts to define what a woman should be, it needs to be challenged.

Women should try to find a new relationship with images. Being depressed because you've failed to live up to an unrealistic ideal is not fair on you. Don't be constrained by stereotyped images. Break out of them and challenge them. Women need greater freedom of choice in discovering how they want to be. Images can be used creatively to express different aspects of being a woman. And how a woman changes over time. After all, there really shouldn't be one right way for women to be.

WHAT YOU CAN DO TO CHANGE YOUR SELF-IMAGE

Join a women's group and talk about your feelings. Go to a counsellor or therapist and talk about how you might redefine your images. Or grab a friend – someone on the same wavelength as you – and discuss how you might change your thinking about yourself.

Learn to be kinder to yourself. Remember, it doesn't matter what media images convey, no woman is 'perfect'. Accept yourself as you are – your imperfect you. That's the first step to stopping that blue feeling – that image-conscious depression which gets you down.

Make peace with all your images – after all, you're a complex woman, and you deserve to have many sides to you. Some of these sides will be individual and some common to all women. Revel in your uniqueness. Enjoy your womanness. And never feel you should be like any other woman.

4

THE CHALLENGE OF RELATIONSHIPS

*Love involves a peculiar unfathomable
combination of understanding and misunderstanding.*

DIANE ARBUS

Myrna Weissman, the prominent researcher into women and depression has said that the majority of women complaining of depression report difficulties in their relationships with spouses and partners. Perhaps this is not surprising, given the emphasis that is placed on the central role of relationships in women's lives.

However, research evidence about women, relationships and depression is complex and contradictory. Many research studies have found that marriage tends to increase women's chances of developing depression, while the opposite happens for men. That is, married men suffer depression less frequently than those who are single or separated. It's been suggested that stereotypes of femininity and the expected role of 'homemaker', even when the woman works outside the home, have contributed to women's greater frequency of depression. Something about married life, or maybe even long-term relationships increases a woman's chances of getting depressed.

Yet, other research, especially case studies and clinical presentations to helping professionals, suggests that single women also are vulnerable to an experience of depression. It seems that if you're a woman then you can't win! Being in a long-term relationship might expose you to depression, but then the single life also might make you more vulnerable.

Perhaps the complexity and contradiction of these findings can be related to the fact that only those women who are depressed by their relationships or, lack of relationships, seek help. Women also are more likely to admit to feelings of dissatisfaction in relationships when they are surveyed in the community. So, at least part of the explanation is that women, whether in relationships, or single, are more prone to discussing their distress, dissatisfaction and other psychological issues. This tendency is a product of women's socialisation, which places a high value on her ability to show emotions and have insight into her psyche. On the other hand, men are socialised to contain their emotions, and a stigma is attached to men emoting too freely.

SOCIETY'S MESSAGES ABOUT THE IMPORTANCE OF RELATIONSHIPS

Pick up any women's magazine, and you'll be confronted by several articles about relationships. Women are given messages that it's wise to develop, keep and work on their relationships in order to achieve happiness. Witness the cover story headlines from recent magazines: 'How to put fun back into your relationship', 'Equal relationships that work: six real-life stories', 'How to seduce any man and make him yours', 'Dumped for another woman: How I got my husband to beg me to take him back', 'Where to meet a man: we road test the places where you're most likely to succeed', 'How to get him back from her bed', 'Would you forgive his adultery?', and 'He still hasn't asked you out? How to make it happen'.

The common thread in many such articles about women and relationships is that women should assume a disproportionate responsibility for finding and then maintaining relationships. The message then is clear: women who experience relationship problems are personal failures. A woman's value is measured in relation to the success (or failure) of her relationships.

Interestingly, women's magazines for the younger market appear to stress the benefits of single status. There are articles and advertising features which appear to show the superior status of being single. However, the message is contradictory. Many competing articles, trumpeting the delights of relationships, appear to overturn the 'single and carefree' ideology.

Rising to the challenge of relationships is a task most women prescribe themselves. They feel responsible to make things happen, to make things work. They strive to find a meaningful relationship. They attempt to patch up ailing relationships. They confront the conflict, disappointments, frustrations and dissatisfactions that are an inevitable part of maintaining any meaningful relationship. This can be exhausting work.

At one level, women have bought the message that making relationships work is women's work. Women have internalised society's message. And often to their cost.

THE MAN/WOMAN THING

Women like chatting. Many men don't. A client, Elaine, once told me that it depressed her that her husband, an otherwise wonderful man did not see the value of chatting – about friends, family, themselves and their relationship. She could have spent hours analysing matters after a dinner party or a family get-together. He simply was not interested in what he considered 'gossip' and often accused her of 'getting into things too deeply'. Not only that, she was hurt and depressed that he hadn't said 'I love you' for years. When she confronted him about this, he said matter-of-factly, 'Of course I love you. I'm still here aren't I?' This was not the response she'd hoped for.

We discussed Elaine's options. Relationship counselling had failed as her husband refused to attend. Elaine had a bright idea. She came up with her own effective solution. It was one that needed constant reapplication, but worked. Elaine didn't want to leave her husband. She just needed to feel she could chat about him in safety. Elaine said that after speaking to me about this issue and having lunch with a friend shortly after – a friend who was a confidant – she was prepared to deal with her husband for the next few months. Elaine clearly felt under great pressure to talk and once she did so, she felt better.

FOR WHOM THE BELL TOLLS

Mae West, in one of her famous one-liners once said: *'Marriage is a great institution, but I'm not ready for an institution yet'.*

Most of us try it at least once in our lives. But marriage might seriously damage your healthy relationship – especially if you're a woman. Remember that research evidence says marriage increases a woman's chances of developing depression.

Wedding guests sometimes murmur darkly about the prospects for the happy couple's future if they marry after years of living together amicably. Why should this be so? Is there any qualitative difference between marriage and merely living together?

Until the 1970s there were good reasons for a couple to get married. Socially accepted sex only happened within marriage and so did children. Practically, the woman needed financial security and the man needed a wife to service his life. But social evolution and the sexual revolution changed all that. These days people can have all the sex and children they want outside marriage – and without much disapproval. A job and a salary provide opportunities for women and a choice of whether or not to manage alone. On the other hand, most men can iron a shirt now.

These changes have made it hard for the couple living together in harmony to make the decision to get married. I know of three cases where couples have lived together for 10 years or more, then married, only to have the marriage last less than one year. Strange but true. Why is this so?

Marriage changes things. It changes the relationship. The views of the world outside start to impinge on your awareness of yourself as part of a couple. People have a different view of a cohabiting couple and a married couple. These outside views apply pressure. A married woman is less likely to be invited out on her own, even on a girls' night out. A married woman can no longer indulge in meaningless flirtations, so good for the ego, because the wedding band reminds her she is spoken for. A married woman is still expected to be an accessory – at her husband's side at functions. The cohabiting woman, on the other hand, is still welcome on a girls' night out, can boost her ego by flirting if the mood takes her and is not expected to accompany her man to that business function.

The outside world impinges on you when you're married. Instead of being treated as an individual sharing a home with another individual, suddenly you're treated as a spouse. Inevitably, you start to see yourself differently. You start to adjust. Marriage, after all, means adjustment. But maybe these adjustments offend you. Maybe you want to remain an individual. Losing your independence might trigger a depression.

One client, Jennifer, described the shifts in her status from live-in lover to wife in financial terms. For her, money was the metaphor for change. She said:

'I've always earned my own money. When we lived together, we had separate accounts and split everything down the middle. Then when we got married, my husband wanted me to relinquish my independence and have a joint account. He talked about 'our' money – suddenly I started to feel like I was being taken over. Other people have said I make too much of this, that it's normal and all that. But for me, it was unacceptable. I got depressed. Did this mean that I'd have to go without something because we needed a new refrigerator, for example? It seemed like I was no longer my own person, I was part of an 'our' situation. I hadn't expected it and I resented it. I told my husband so – that I refused to be so controlled. It took ages to sort this out. I now have my own account and I agreed to a small joint account.'

Jennifer is lucky. She earns her own money and was strong enough to insist on some ground rules regarding shared finances, which she could live with. Other women are not so lucky. They either become financially dependent on their husbands or feel coerced into joint funds which represent their loss of financial independence. It's easy to see how such a loss can trigger a depression. The woman feels powerless and trapped.

A friend of mine once said that after living with her partner for eleven years and then marrying him, life changed inexplicably. Suddenly she felt she belonged to some sort of club, the membership of which changed her relationship. She said:

'Once I took my vows, my relationship, my marriage seemed to become public property, in a way I'd never experienced before. My intentions even became

public property. Suddenly, colleagues and even complete strangers seemed to think it okay to ask when I was going to have children. It was amazing.'

Sometimes, the trials of marriage are just enough to test the strength and resilience of love. If the relationship is shaky, then making it legal is unlikely to magically improve the quality of the relationship.

A psychologist friend who works with battling couples on the verge of separation and divorce sometimes sits and wonders. She tells me that she often finds herself confronted by couples consumed by enormous amounts of hostility, resentment and depression. Sometimes she asks herself the simple question: 'Why on earth did these people get married in the first place?'

Or perhaps the question should be: 'What went wrong?'

PAIN IN RELATIONSHIPS

Of course, relationships can be a celebration of life and all things good and positive. Equally, they can cause much pain and at times, utter despair. Pleasure and pain – the flip sides of the coin.

William Shakespeare once wrote:
'The course of true love never did run smooth'.
Indeed.

Many women think that men should be more like their women friends. A common argument develops when the woman demands the same response from her man as she gets from her woman friends. Men secretly wish that their women should, to quote Professor Higgins in *My Fair Lady*, – 'be more like a man.' Given these different expectations from relationships, it's reasonable to assume that true love rarely runs smoothly – and if it does, it means that both parties are working to make it so.

Often, it's the woman who's taking charge of improving the relationship. Take the case of Amy, a 35 year old woman who works as a beauty therapist and is the mother of one girl aged 9. She believes she has the 'best of both worlds' and she's content with her arrangement of family and career.

However, she's unhappy about her husband's emotional absence from their relationship. She says:

> 'I don't think I expect too much from Mike. But, of course, he thinks I do. It's too much to expect him to be civil when he comes home from work, it's too much to ask him to help around the place and it's definitely too much to ask him to pay attention, to listen to what I have to say. He tells me he's tired and wants to relax – well, what about me? – I work too but I try to make our relationship work.
>
> 'He's so distant – not only with me, but with Katie as well. Sometimes I get so depressed about it. I don't know what to do. We've been for counselling, but he kind of boycotts it and he just says, 'men are different' – like a joke, only he really means it. I try so hard to communicate, but I get so little back from him. Sometimes I think I'm burning myself out.'

Amy goes on to say that before they married she thought he'd change. She wanted to believe that maybe he'd become a 'sensitive new age guy'.

Along with countless other women before her, Amy subscribed to the idea that: 'Women hope men will change after marriage but they don't. Men hope women won't change but they do.'

Doris, a 42 year old teacher admits to believing her ex-husband would change. She thought that once they married, they'd become a close, intimate couple, able to share thoughts, feelings and secrets freely and easily. Her experience proved her expectations wrong. She comments:

> 'My marriage was going to be a perfect one. I married late-ish – at 34 – and I'd held out to find what I considered an almost perfect partner. I guess my expectations were pretty high – that's why it took me to 34 to find him!
>
> 'But even then it didn't work out as I'd imagined. David and I shared all sorts of things in common. He was good-looking and charming and I thought a real catch! There was an emotional hardness about him – but I thought I could polish that side of him up a bit. Two years into our marriage and he wasn't any softer – if anything – he seemed to have toughened up in response to my attempts to get him to be more caring, gentle and understanding.
>
> 'I guess I needed a man who could nurture me and David couldn't. I got really very depressed in the last year of our relationship – we were together for

five years – because I felt I wasn't getting anything from him. He was walled off to me. We had sex and that was good at times – we're both quite physical – but I needed more – much more. I needed to be cuddled and held and told how much I was loved. David wasn't demonstrative like that. I think he was frightened of letting go and being soft and caring. There was no real communication between us.'

Communication. A simple word with many complex meanings. Its most commonly used meaning refers to the exchange of words between people. Talking.

Research has found that women and men have different ideas about talking. For women, the purpose generally is to get closer to people, without having any specific goal in mind. But for men, talking usually is about exchanging information. The process of talking is important for women. Men like the bottom line – they like to get to the point.

Not surprisingly, research also has found that women are good at talking about their feelings to women friends. They've been doing it since they were girls. Men don't have that experience.

Generally speaking, women are good at communication. They give non-verbal signals when listening to others. They are sensitive to paying attention to what the other person is saying. Women regularly talk to each other about their personal, inner lives.

Asking men to talk – to communicate – as women do, means helping them learn a new language. It's a little difficult and it takes a long time. Defeat, burnout and depression sometimes are reached before the new communication patterns develop. Women sometimes give up on men and their relationships.

SOME INTERESTING INFORMATION

Studies have shown a real gender difference in communication. Women when listening are much more likely to give what are called 'minimal encouragers' – making sounds like 'yeah', 'uh-huh' and 'mmm' which indicate they are listening and following what is being said. Men, on the other hand, are more likely to remain silent. This is why many women complain their partners never listen while the men protest that they've heard every word.

A friend who was frustrated with her partner's silence, has taken to asking him to repeat what she's said – particularly important information, to assure herself that he has listened.

Other non-verbal signals can also indicate whether your partner is tuned in. Watch for eye contact, facial expression and subtle bodily gestures.

CIRCLE THIS

Don't forget that conversation is a mutual exchange of ideas and information. When you find yourself speaking without feedback, you get the feeling you're talking to a wall. Help your partner – if he's the silent type – to give some feedback so you won't have to wonder if he's really listening.

LOVE DOES NOT CONQUER ALL

Loving someone does not automatically equip you to deal with a difficult relationship situation. Take the case of adultery. Endless numbers of words of advice are dispensed yearly in women's magazines about what to do if you find your partner in another woman's arms. But what happens when it really happens?

Laura is one woman whose husband's adultery meant the end of their relationship and the beginning of her six-month depression. Laura is a 26 year old woman who works in a part-time clerical position. She had been married for 3 years and has an eighteen month old son, Jesse. Laura came home unexpectedly one day to find her husband in bed with another woman. After much soul-searching she decided to leave her husband. She says:

'It was like something out of a bad movie and I can still see it in my mind's eye. I don't think I'll ever be able to shake that image – you hear about this sort of thing happening, you read about it but who would've thought it would happen to me? I thought I had a marriage made in heaven.

'Bob was big, strong, good-looking and very sensitive. Even after Jesse was born, Bob was romantic, surprising me with little things, buying me sexy lingerie, boxes of chocolates, who knows, maybe he did all of that because he

had a guilty conscience. All my friends were jealous of me thinking I had it all – and I thought I did until that day.

'Bob was the most wonderful husband a woman could ask for – so attentive, warm and loving. We had ourselves a ball. Sex was good but after Jesse came along I got a touch of the baby blues and Bob and I argued a little. I was tired a lot of the time, but I still gave him lots of attention. Clearly it wasn't enough because – it's a cliche – he found solace in the arms of another woman. How many times has this story been told I wonder?

'As it happened, I found out by pure chance. Bob was on night shift and said he'd mind Jesse while I went to a pottery class. Normally I take Jesse with me or I drop him off at a friend's place. That day I took Bob up on his offer and went to my class. But I wasn't feeling well so I came home a few hours early to find Bob in our bed with another woman. Jesse was in the next room in his play-pen while they were having sex.

'I can tell you I could have killed them both. I went mad and they both looked scared. Unfortunately, Jesse was upset by the scene and cried and cried. He was as inconsolable as I felt. After I hounded the woman out, Bob and I had a real battle. By this time I'd taken Jesse to a neighbour's place. I couldn't see him upset. What really infuriated me was that Bob tried to justify his behaviour. He said I had made him feel unloved and that he had felt the need to prove he was still attractive. I couldn't believe his arrogance. What a selfish and cruel man, I kept thinking. He was having an affair and trying to pin the blame on me.'

For Laura, the betrayal of trust and sense of rejection caused her to become depressed. She chose to end the relationship, because the pain of continuing, and not knowing, would prove to be too much. In her case, love couldn't conquer all.

FEAR AND LOVING

Nor could love conquer all in the case of Stella. She is a 50 year old woman who has been divorced for five years. For 20 out of the 25 years of her marriage she alternated between fear and loving – two emotions which her husband raised in equal parts in her. She comments:

'To the outside world, my husband was this charming, sophisticated man. He was a television producer and did an excellent job. I'm told that at work he was a saint. But it was a different picture at home.

'Much of the time he was a loving husband and kind father, but then he'd have fits of rage and the children and I would cower and fear for our lives. He wasn't a drinker. That's the strange thing – there was never any escalation of violence – we didn't know when to expect it – he'd just snap. Sometimes he'd snap over silly, little things – it was very difficult to take. He only hit the kids on a couple of occasions – I think his strength and rage frightened even him. I think he thought he might've killed them. But with me, it was a different story. He wasn't as scared of hitting me.

'I used to get very depressed, thinking it was all my fault. I went to see my doctor once, but he was so shocked when I told him, I felt sorry for him! We both pretended it didn't happen.

'Then, after years of putting up with it and feeling so lonely and depressed – I thought I'd die of shame if I let anyone I knew really well, know. Anyway, one night after we came home from a dinner party, without saying a word, he hit me across the face. I fell back against the wall and hit my head badly. I had a very bad cut lip. My husband told me he was teaching me a lesson for contradicting him in public. I felt devastated. That night I decided to leave him. But I had to think of the kids – so it took another six years before I left. In the meantime, I'd gone to a mental health centre and was getting counselling – in secret – I couldn't let him know. I think that counseling gave me the strength to eventually leave him.'

Statistics reveal that domestic violence occurs in one of five relationships. Domestic violence is evidence of a relationship gone very wrong. However, rates based on records are probably underestimates of the real situation. Usually only the more severe cases of domestic violence are brought to official attention. In terms of the actual events, the most frequent types of violence experienced by women include grabbing, shoving, pushing, slapping, kicking, biting and hitting with a fist.

Some women find themselves at their doctor's offices complaining of anxiety and depression. Often they are too embarrassed to admit to the abuse. If they have physical signs of injury they will concoct a half-believable story. The reality is too much to bear at times. When you live with unbelievable fear of a man you once loved – and maybe still love – the likelihood of getting depressed is high.

Contrary to popular belief, domestic violence is not confined to a certain class or group of people. As Stella's account shows, an otherwise well-respected, likeable man can have a dark, secret side, known only to his family.

I was working in a community health center when Briony came to see me. She was an attractive, vivacious woman of 38, who had a history of depressions and attempted suicides. Her physician had referred her for therapy, suspecting, quite rightly, that Briony wasn't telling him everything.

It took about six weeks before Briony was able to begin trusting me with the intimate details of her life – a life of emotional abuse and regular beatings. Briony worked as a high school teacher and her husband was an attorney. They had been married for ten years and had two children, aged 7 and 5.

Cautiously, little by little, Briony began to tell me what it was like to be her – to live in a state torn between terrible fear and great love of her husband. Her story reinforces the fact that an abuser, a batterer, isn't who you think he is. Briony told me she was attracted to Graham in the first instance because he was attractive, warm, charming and loving. Briony believed him when he said he loved her bubbliness, her intelligence, her beauty. Briony thought it was a match made in heaven. Then about six months into their marriage, all hell broke loose. It started without warning. Briony said she suddenly couldn't do anything right. She couldn't please Graham.

But it wasn't always darkness. At times, Graham was apologetic, wanting to talk, buying her gifts, pretending everything was normal. Briony's life alternated between darkness and light. She lived in hope. She told herself things would get better. She told herself Graham would change. She rationalised his behaviour – he'd had a terrible childhood. She became anxious living with him. She didn't know when he'd strike. Then she became depressed. She took some sleeping tablets and cut her wrists. But she still didn't tell anyone about her private hell. She was too ashamed.

For years, Graham would come home from work and take out his frustrations on Briony. He would ring her from the office and tell her to prepare herself for a beating. He beat her in front of the children. He forced her to have sex every night, often waking her at all hours and if she resisted, he'd wake the children and then beat her into submission. He prided himself on being smart and told her no-one would believe her story. He often hit her in the stomach, where the damage wouldn't show. When she was visibly bruised she learned to tell plausible stories. People seemed to believe her – perhaps people wanted to believe her. She became a clumsy person – a klutz. He threatened her that if she told anyone, went to the police, he would cut her throat. But the final straw came when he made her kneel in front of him and beg his forgiveness, while he stood over her with a large knife.

It was shortly after that episode that Briony went to her doctor, complaining of depression – and she was referred to me. Briony was suffering anxiety, depression and low self-esteem. It was difficult for Briony to reveal so much of her 'shame' to me. I was respectful towards her and encouraged her to free herself of the guilt and shame she felt. We worked on exploring her options, emotionally and legally. Within four months of coming to see me, Briony knew she had to leave the abuse behind.

I remember her words clearly. She said, *'Thank you for helping me break the silence. It had become such a burden.'*

Having your partner circle you like a shark and give you a necklace of bruises is unacceptable. Domestic violence is a mind game. It's a psychological thriller where the woman as victim loses all sense of what's rational and what's irrational. But leaving is difficult, because the woman often wants to believe that things will get better. Until she becomes so depressed that she attempts to take her life – and then part of her knows she must leave – sooner or later.

Some women find themselves in the victim role in relationships. Of course, not all women who feel like victims in their relationships are battered. Sometimes this sense of victimhood is psychological. They find themselves depressed and with little self-esteem. They wonder what love really is and if it's worth the anxiety and depression of staying in a relationship.

Diane Harpwood in her amusing book ***Tea and Tranquillizers*** has her heroine record the following in her diary:

> *'Sunday 22nd. I doubt if love exists. It's just a word used to describe a violent emotion that bursts into fiery life in adolescence and dies quietly with maturity – like acne. It's mother nature's con-trick, necessary to ensure the survival of the species, the pairing and mating. But, once we've paired and mated, love is redundant. What then? Is there love after marriage? Love is just a euphemism for sex.'*

But what about expectations? Is it the case that some women expect too much from their relationships? This idea of expectations and the mismatch that occurs between men and women in relationships where there is a communication breakdown signals the death of emotions, of that bonding which is sometimes called 'love'.

THE SOUNDS OF SILENCE

As Olivia is telling me her story of dashed hopes, failed expectations and frank depression, I'm reminded of the Simon and Garfunkel song, The Sounds of Silence.

Olivia, 52, a woman best described as outgoing and vital, tells me that her depression, stemming from the lack of life in her relationship, was reinforced for years by her friends and her mother. They all told her she was expecting too much. While Olivia's world was experienced as 'echoes to the sound of silence', her mother was telling her, '*You have to learn to live with it my dear. That's just the way men are. They're not capable of talking about things like we are*'. Olivia became depressed and lost all hope of having what she calls 'an equal relationship'. She met a blank wall and she accepted it. This acceptance came at the cost of her feelings of depression.

The 'sounds of silence' syndrome is a complaint of many depressed women. One client told me, '*Okay, I like him strong, but the silent bit really gets to me. I used to exhaust myself by trying to get him to open up. Now I just accept that that's the way he is.'*

It's easy to see how a couple can lapse into silence. Because if Jane asks John every evening: 'How was your day?' and John replies with 'Fine, how was yours?' then a certain pattern develops. Unless one of them breaks the pattern, this couple will stop communicating except in the most superficial way. Maybe Jane can't be bothered to pursue further communication. Perhaps she's tried before but John has erected a wall of silence.

One experienced therapist says that the sounds of silence are set up in our sex-role conditioning. She believes that boys are brought up to express almost nothing except anger, to be dominant and achieving and to show leadership skills. This means that it's almost impossible to 'be emotional'. That prescription is given to girls. The logic goes as follows: If you are emotional, you can't be rational. However, it's time to ask: Is expressing emotion irrational?

Expressing emotions and opening up can enhance communication. But sometimes, it's hard for a couple, set in poor communication patterns, to regain the intimacy that is communication's gift. Women are not, of course, solely responsible for the quality of communication in a relationship. But often, they assume that role as a result of their conditioning. There are men who find it hard to express their emotions and to respond to the woman's efforts to bring them out emotionally. In such cases, she gives up and becomes depressed.

It's true to say that communication is important for a relationship. Learning to understand one another can make a big difference in how you feel about your relationship and yourself. Lara, a woman who had been referred to me for depression says she learned to 'really listen, show attention' and then taught her husband to do the same.

Follow Lara's example by learning to understand how you might better communicate your thoughts and feelings. Practise your communication skills. When you feel empowered enough, teach your partner how he might communicate better.

> **Exercise** **Practising better communication skills**
>
> Communication skills are fundamental to relating to others. They include all the verbal and non-verbal ways we can express our thoughts and feelings. Without clear communication from you, others may not understand your low mood and this can put a strain on the relationship. Remember the following points:
>
> - Tell people how you feel, clearly and constructively
> - Correct any mistaken assumptions or guesses others have made
> - Don't send contradictory messages, for example, don't say 'I'm okay' when everything about you says you're not
> - Don't have others guessing about you. For example, if your non-verbal message to others is that you obviously feel bad, but you say nothing about it, then you are sending two messages. The first is that you feel bad, but the second is that you don't want to talk about it. That makes the people around you guess at what's wrong, and often leaves them confused.

Even if you have good social skills, when you've got the blues, you're probably not using them. By getting in touch with your coping social skills and developing new ones, you'll be able to control your moods much better.

Being able to communicate effectively and to stand up for your feelings and rights are essential to gaining control of your emotions and life. Learning to express feelings before they build up and become overwhelming helps you stay in control. Don't stew on things. Deal with problems and grievances as they arise.

HOW TO SHARE YOUR FEELINGS CONSTRUCTIVELY

1. LEARN TO 'LEVEL' ABOUT YOUR FEELINGS

You can level by simply announcing your feelings and what you think might have triggered them. For example: 'You know, I've been remembering what happened to me and now I feel real down'.

If the trigger for your blues was the behaviour of another person, something that he or she did that triggered your feelings, then you level with an X-Y-Z statement. This X-Y-Z formula is a constructive way to communicate your feelings: 'When you did X, the effect on me was Y and I felt Z.'

Example:
'When you tell me to forget about what happened to me, it stops me from telling you how I really feel, and I feel even worse.'

Levelling with the X-Y-Z formula tells the other person exactly what he or she did, how it affected you, and how you feel about it. You'll find that it's a most effective way of sharing strong feelings within any relationship.

At first, you might find this awkward. But, with practice, it becomes a natural way of sharing important feelings.

Let's break it down, one part at a time.

'When you do X...'
This should be a simple statement, describing the other person's behaviour. For example: 'When you put me down in front of others...'

- Don't make vague statements like, 'When you do things that remind my of my boss...' because then the other person has to guess what he or she has done that reminded you of your boss.
- Don't level with interpretations, like 'You don't really care how I feel...' because the other person has to guess which part of their behaviour seems uncaring to you.
- Don't overgeneralise, like, 'You always put me down...' Overgeneralisations are rarely true and they invite the other person to look for the exception. This can lead into avoiding your original concern.
- Don't assassinate the other person's character, like, 'You're just a mean, uncaring person...' because the other person again has to guess what they have done to give you that impression. They will probably be defensive about what they see as an overwhelming condemnation.

'...the effect on me is Y...'
This should be a brief, clear description of how the other person's behaviour directly affects you. It has been found that if you tell people how you've

been directly affected by their behaviour, they pay more attention to your levelling. They also may be more willing to change their behaviour.

Continuing the example: 'When you put me down in front of others, that reminds me of my boss's attitude…'

Now, the other person is aware of exactly how his or her behaviour has affected you and may be more willing to change it.

- Don't order or threaten, like, 'You must not do that anymore, or I'll leave.' Orders and threats don't work as most people resent this sort of treatment.
- Don't moralise or lecture, like, 'You ought to be more sensitive to my feelings.' By moralising, you're saying that your morals are superior to the other person's. Usually, this offends people and lessens your influence with them.
- Don't level on the wrong issue, like, 'You're showing what a brute you are…' when your real concern is that you are being put down and how it reminds you of your boss's attitude towards you.

'…And I feel Z'

This should be a clear and accurate statement of your feelings.

Continuing the example: 'When you put me down in front of others, that reminds me of my boss's attitude and I feel belittled and angry.'

Be as accurate as you can be about the strength of your feelings. If you were feeling angry rather than irritated, then you should say 'angry'.

- Don't try to keep your feelings to yourself by leaving out the Z part of your levelling statement. You may feel a little embarrassed at first, but remember that to share your feelings constructively, you must take risks.
- Don't blame others for your feelings with you-statements like, '…you make me feel so awful.' Other people are not responsible for your feelings. While their actions may influence how you feel, you are in control of how you think and what you do in response.
- Don't weaken your levelling, like, '…I feel a little upset', when you feel very angry. If you make the situation seem unimportant to you, that's how the other person sees it too.

- Don't zap back, trying to hurt the other person because you've been hurt, like 'You might think I'm being silly but you're just an insensitive brute, without an ounce of thoughtfulness in your body.' You may feel tempted to zap back, if you think the other person has hurt you, but it will give you only short-term satisfaction. Your communication will be more effective if you level rather than zap. Levelling is more constructive than zapping.

- Don't level only about bad feelings. Level about good feelings as well as bad ones, like 'I'm feeling a lot better today' or 'When we talk about how I feel when you put me down I am grateful you're so open and honest with me.' By telling someone what they did to make you feel better, you'll increase the chances of that happening again.

Exercise **Now it's your turn**

Think about levelling. Work out some levelling statements you could use to tell important people in your life about strong feelings that are triggered by parts of their behaviour.

Use the X-Y-Z formula – 'When you did X, the effect on me was Y and I felt Z.' Practice your levelling statements in your imagination and take the next chance to use them in real life.

2. ASKING FOR CHANGES IN BEHAVIOUR

Sometimes it's enough for you to level about your strong feelings. At other times, it isn't enough to share your feelings because you also want some change in the situation. This happens when your strong feelings have been triggered by the other person's behaviour and you would like to see a change. The most effective way to get someone to consider changing their behaviour is to make a request. However, making requests is not easy. You may feel reluctant to make a request.

For instance, 'I couldn't ask him to do that...' 'She might get angry...' or 'He should know how I feel...' These are poor reasons for not asking for what you want. The first reason suggests that you think people have to accept your requests. In fact, you can make a request and they have the right to refuse. The second one implies that you can't cope if someone gets angry with you. The third says that other people should be mind-readers. Don't leave anything to guesswork.

Your requests need to be clear and precise to be effective. The other person has to know exactly what you want.

- effective requests are for observable behaviour, so that you know when it's happened
- effective requests are made in positive and non-defensive terms, quietly and politely, but firmly
- effective requests have a positive content, which means that you're asking the other person to do something that you want, not to stop doing something that you don't want

Remember your body language. When making a request, try to have some eye-contact and speak clearly.

Exercise Practise, practise, practise

Stop and think about some requests you can make to important people in your life. Follow the guidelines above and look at the examples below. At first, practise making your requests in your imagination and then look for chances to use them in real life.

Some better alternatives to bad requests

Some bad requests	Some better alternatives
'I want you to show you really understand' (too vague)	'I would like you to ask me how I am feeling and listen to what I say'
'I want you to quit telling me how I feel' (too negative)	'Please accept that I know my own feelings
'I want some support!' (too vague)	'I would really like us to sit down and talk about this crisis I'm facing'

A helpful hint

If you feel uncertain about levelling and making requests, try to practise them in your imagination first. Then you can work on some of these techniques with a trusted person, with whom you have a good relationship. Doing some role-play exercises with that person, trying out your skills in levelling and making requests, provides you with a safe environment in which to practise. Once you feel comfortable in these practice sessions, you will be more likely to remember how to use the skills when strong feelings occur in other situations.

('Levelling' and the 'X-Y-Z' Formula: adapted from Montgomery & Morris, 1989.)

While some married women ask about the cost of love, sex and relationships, there are single women who enviously wish to have all three, regardless of the costs. Or so they think.

THE SINGLE LIFE AS DEPRESSANT

'All my single years, it seems to me, consisted of fifteen minutes of perfect rapture and fifteen weeks of perfect misery.': Judith Viorst in **Yes, Married**.

Every woman is single at some time. Times have changed and today, it's more acceptable for women to remain single. In fact, 18% of all American women over eighteen are single. But while it is far more acceptable for women to remain single today than even 20 years ago, society's view of the single woman contributes towards depression.

Dinah, a 36 year old lawyer sums it up well in her statement, *'People still view the single woman, especially the ageing single woman, as a reject. No matter what I accomplish, I don't have status in some people's eyes – I've failed to pair up with a man.'*

But however 'modern' some single women are in their views and desire for independence, there are as many others who are searching for a meaningful relationship. 'Meeting someone' and 'having a relationship' are high on the agenda of many single women.

Dorothy Parker, writer and wit, wrote a compelling short story almost 50 years ago. It is a story about a woman waiting anxiously by the telephone. She is prepared to sell her soul to the devil, if only her man would ring. The heroine says:

> *'Please, God, let him telephone me now. Dear God let him call me now. I won't ask anything else of You, truly I won't. It isn't very much to ask. It would be so little to You, God, such a little, little thing. Only let him telephone now. Please, God. Please, please, please.'*

She then bargains with herself, challenges herself to not ring her lover, and believes that God is punishing her as the phone remains silent. She wants to play the dating game correctly and adopts a seemingly rational approach:

> *'I won't. I'll be quiet. This is nothing to get excited about. Look. Suppose he were someone I didn't know very well. Suppose he were another girl. Then I'd just telephone and say, 'Well, for goodness' sake, what happened to you?' That's what I'd do, and I'd never even think about it. Why can't I be casual and natural, just because I love him? I can be. Honestly, I can be. I'll call him up, and be so easy and pleasant. You see if I won't, God. Oh, don't let me call him. Don't, don't, don't.'*

All these years later, there are many single women who can identify with Parker's heroine. They can identify with the anguish and pain of being single and waiting to be phoned for a date.

Women report confusion. There is still heavy-duty confusion around who is supposed to call, to invite out and to pay. The etiquette and rules of the single life and dating game are no clearer today than yesterday. For many single women, the dating game, the quest for a relationship, often ends in dating fatigue and depression. One wit said, 'Dating is more stressful than prison'.

Leigh, 38, a pharmacist, was quoted in Chapter One as saying that 'men are the cause of a lot of depression among women'. Leigh is a quietly spoken woman who has been married for over a year now. I ask her to elaborate on her theory. She says:

> *'I was single for a long time. I dated a lot and I found men so frustrating and difficult. A lot of men have some 'dream woman' image in their heads – they pitch their expectations too high or unrealistically. A lot of men – more than I ever imagined – want some Barbie-doll type woman, sweet and pretty.*

> 'Dating was like a duel instead of a dance for me. I'm a fairly confident woman and that seemed to threaten many men. I wanted to be accepted on equal terms and many men find that impossible. I think younger women have a terrible time – a depressing time – being single and dating is no fun. You're made to feel vulnerable. You live with the constant fear of rejection.
>
> 'A wonderful friend, who's 32 rang me in tears the other day. She looks great but was told by one sleazy guy who, although educated, leered and groped, but when she sent him packing, he abused her for being a 'feminist' whose legs were not long enough and whose thighs are too big. That's what I mean by men being a cause of a lot of depression. I rest my case.'

Leigh tells me that before she settled down with her husband, her 18 year dating career was beginning to take on the spectre of gladiatorial combat. Men and the quest for a meaningful relationship were making her feel very depressed.

Finding yourself suddenly single can also lead to depression. A widowed client, Ruth, 49, told me that being single and learning the dating code was anxiety-provoking and depressing. After 28 years of marriage, she was struggling to relearn the ground rules, and she had approached a romance broker as a final quick-fix solution. Not only did she part with lots of hard cash, but her three 'introductions' were disappointing. Eventually she joined a ballroom dancing class and after a few go-nowhere dates, she decided to adopt a no-nonsense line. She says that being assertive helped her over her feelings of depression – powerlessness and feelings of rejection. She says:

> 'I was tired of the silly games and analysing every contact with a potential partner. I decided I wasn't going to wonder and worry about if he'd ring me. I was up-front and said, 'Call me if you're interested'.

'Call me if you're interested' – is a very powerful message. It's also one that means that Ruth didn't have to wait by the phone like Parker's heroine. Ruth's simple message conveys her interest, but not desperation and leaves the decision to the man. This suits her. Ruth wasn't expecting a phone call, and she had put herself in the unambiguous position of not having to become neurotic and depressed if that phone call never came. However, if she does get the phone call she knows he is interested.

The dating game and the search for a relationship can become all-consuming for some women. When the search becomes so intensified, it begins to take on the proportions of an obsession. And obsessions can be depressing.

Pamela is 39, and has always managed musicians. She's enjoyed her work and had little time for a permanent relationship – until now. Recently, she found herself feeling low, something which was new to her. She fears that her search for a relationship has become too important. That depresses her. She says:

> 'A friend laughed and told me it wasn't a relationship I wanted, just a baby – tick tock, tick tock... Maybe there's some truth in that – but not entirely. I guess I'm just ready to settle down and there doesn't seem much hope at the moment. 'It's the old story – all the good men are taken – or gay – or both! You know, I didn't think I'd get so depressed about it. After all, I was going to be the eternal single girl, enjoying all my freedom etc. Now I see couples in the supermarket and I get jealous. I can't believe it. It's almost pathetic. In fact, I seem to see couples all around me all the time. It's like the rest of the world is flaunting being a pair – and here I am this pathetic, single, ageing woman. I think it's time I went to an introduction agency or did one of those voice-mail numbers – here I am, lonely and depressed, come and get me! I didn't think I'd ever get this down about not having a committed relationship. Just goes to show how your attitude changes with time.'

Pamela knows she must watch herself and her new obsession. It could take over her life. She sums it up well when she says:

> 'I'm basically a fairly balanced person and I'm not going to let this search for Mr. Right destroy my life. A little depression is one thing but I can't let myself be crippled by it.'

Pamela's caution about being 'crippled' by the overwhelming need to find a relationship and the depression that results, is a wise one. Yet, the drive to find a partner is strong within us and encouraged by society. Everywhere you look, there are romance brokers offering the opportunity of a relationship. But the sort of chemistry which makes for a good relationship is deeper than the sort of superficial compatibility of *'I like Mozart, movies, moonlight strolls and dining alfresco'*.

A good friend who found herself single after fifteen years of a 'so-so' relationship says: *'The worst thing about being single is being single. In a couple-oriented world, being single is like a stigma'*.

Single women are said to be the least depressed of all women. However, like every generalisation, it has its exceptions. Singlehood does not suit every woman. For every woman who is content with being single, there is probably another, like Leigh, Ruth and Pamela, who is increasingly dissatisfied and depressed. And possibly feeling stigmatised.

Many single women complain that they feel they don't belong. If they've been in a relationship which has ended, they suddenly find they have stopped being invited out by friends. These friends may be motivated by embarrassment and terror of being accused either of taking sides or of matchmaking. One woman who became single again in her forties described to me how she felt like a misfit, even a leper – her former friends studiously avoided her. She added that one friend told her that as a married woman she was 'safe', but as a single woman she was a threat. She laughed as she told me that *'people certainly show their true colours when the chips are down'*.

It's easy to understand how being shunned in times of psychological need, can take its toll. However simplistic it sounds, women who are single should be encouraged to not fall into the trap of believing that they can't be fulfilled unless they are part of a couple.

Interestingly, the women's magazines often run feature articles about the benefits of being single. In the late 1980s and early 1990s there was a glut of such articles. Then it was almost fashionable to be single and celibate. But, from the mid-1990s, the magazines appear to be hedging their bets. Women alternatively, are being told that it's healthy and unhealthy to be single. Articles on offer include: 'The surprising payoffs of being single', 'The life and good times of single women', 'What singles hate about couples' and 'Happiness and the single woman', the latter being an article with mixed messages about the advantages and disadvantages of being female and single.

RELATIONSHIPS – KEEPING THE FAITH

Dorothy Parker, in another of her incisive short stories, titled *'The Sexes'* captures the struggle involved in communicating in relationships. A courting couple are involved in an ever-increasingly complex game of non-communication . . .

"I haven't the faintest idea what you're talking about," she said. "There isn't a thing on earth the matter. I don't know what you mean."

"Yes, you do," he said. "There's something the trouble. Is it anything I've done, or anything?"

"Goodness," she said, "I'm sure it isn't any of my business, anything you do. I certainly wouldn't feel I had any right to criticize."

"Will you stop talking like that?" he said. "Will you, please?"

"Talking like what?" she said.

And so it continues. This struggle with communication. Parker's characters were trying to speak to one another 50 years ago, but equally they could be trying to communicate with each other today.

Relationships. They are a necessary part of our life. They are difficult to get right. They provide all of us with a huge challenge. Sometimes it's hard not to believe that men and women think, feel and act differently. Of course, this can provide variety and spontaneity in relationships. Complementing one another is a good thing. On the other hand, these differences can also lead to conflict, disappointment, unmet needs, loneliness, frustration, anxiety and ultimately, depression.

CHANGING TIMES

Times are changing. Recent statistics highlight that women are moving out of relationships which depress them. In fact, in the United States, up to 75% of divorces are initiated by the woman. The situation in Britain is such that for every man who divorces his wife, three women divorce their husbands. In Australia, it is women rather than men who are deciding to end the marriage. In approximately 65% of cases, it is the woman who makes the decision to separate and divorce. This trend is mirrored in other Western countries.

These statistics imply a shift. Better laws, the women's movement and greater consciousness on the part of women has led to their actions to leave unsatisfactory relationships.

Women's new found financial independence means that more women have greater choices. Relationships are important for us all. Women still seem to believe they should take an unequal responsiblity for making them work. However, when the relationship flounders, women are quicker to exit. This trend is much healthier than the one which kept women in unhappy relationships. Unhappy, powerless and depressed. Relationship depression, at least as far as women are concerned, is being redefined.

MOVING TOWARDS MUTUAL COMMUNICATION

Women's increased awareness and assertiveness has meant they are wanting better quality communication. The men's movement has led many men to an understanding of the importance of mutual communication. However, quality mutual communication cannot take place when the partners are afraid of hearing what the other person has to say – or afraid of really being heard. Both partners must be interested in investing in their relationship. If couples cannot, by themselves, reach a position where both partners believe they can be heard, then couples counselling is an option. By becoming more aware of communication patterns in a relationship – and working towards making communication more effective, fewer women might report relationship difficulties. If Myrna Weissman's observations are correct, this would mean less relationship depression for women.

5
TROUBLE IN THE TEEN YEARS

One of the things I've discovered in general about raising kids is that they really don't give a damn if you walked five miles to school. They want to deal with what's happening now.

PATTY DUKE

'Yes', 'no' and 'don't know' were the three responses Shaylee gave to every question I put to her. At times like that, an hour can seem like an eternity. Shaylee, 14, had been referred by the local high school for counselling because of her 'difficult and unco-operative behaviour'. I was beginning to see the teachers' point of view. Shaylee was proving extremely 'difficult and unco-operative'. It wasn't hard to see how she'd gained those labels. She sat with her head down low, downcast eyes and flat voice conveying her monosyllables. She looked depressed.

Just as the long hour was drawing to a close and almost as if she sensed this, Shaylee looked up and said: 'It's my birthday tomorrow'. When I asked her what she'd most like to do on her birthday, she said unhesitatingly, 'Run away from home'.

Shaylee dropped a bombshell. She also told me in four simple words that she was depressed enough about her life to run from it. Running away from home is something many depressed teenagers do. They hope to run away from their misery and run towards something better. However, they often find that running away means taking your problems to another location. Leaving behind your depression is not that easy.

Being an adolescent – a teenager – can be a trying time. It is a time of changeability. The average teenager can become the veritable Dr Jekyll and Mr. Hyde, experiencing the highest highs and the lowest lows, all in a matter of hours. The word adolescence comes from the Latin word 'adolescere' which means 'to grow up'. This process of growing up takes place between the ages of 13 and 19, which we commonly term the 'teenage' years.

The word 'teenager' was coined during the latter part of the 1940s by market researchers who wanted to describe young people with money to spend. According to one pundit, *'Teenagers were born in 1942, marketed in America in 1947... cosseted and comforted during the 1960s, began to weaken in the 1970s, and can now be pronounced extinct'.*

But each generation brings its own crop of teenagers trying to find themselves and launch themselves into adulthood. In fact, some people have argued that instead of the teenage culture weakening, as the pundit predicted, it's gone from strength to strength. The rise of teenage culture has brought its stresses as well. The teenage years are often referred to as a period of 'storm and stress'.

The storms and stresses of the teenager relate to changes – the impact of biology, changing bodies, roles and expectations. It's a time of emotional instability, mood swings, uncertainties, ambivalence about maturity and separation and the distress of constant self-analysis.

TEEN YEARS: NEGOTIATING THE CHANGES

Teenage years should be filled with carefree laughter, phone calls, parties and convertibles. But the reality is that for many teenagers, the second decade of their life is the most traumatic period of their entire lives.

Physical, social and psychological changes mark the teenage years. These changes of adolescence are rapid and often occur simultaneously. During puberty, girls experience growth in height of approximately 10 inches and a gain of body fat of approximately 24 pounds. For many girls, leaving behind their long, thin, pre-teenage shape is stressful. In an attempt to retain that shape, the shape and lines of their emerging role-models – the supermodels – many teenage girls begin to diet.

In a 1998 survey, 47% of girls between 10 and 17 said that body image was a cause of their stress and depression.

Social changes occur when the teenager moves from the fairly structured, elementary school to a less structured and often large middle or high school. New and more difficult courses require increased self-discipline and decisions regarding future careers need to be faced. Some teenagers also begin working for wages and this can mean less time with friends, new responsibilities, learning to manage money. Another major change for the teenage girl is dating. She starts going out with boys and learning to handle sexual encounters and develop relationships.

Psychological and emotional turmoil is another change to be negotiated. The teenage girl has to negotiate a marked change in physical appearance, leaving behind the childhood sense of herself. Often girls become appearance obsessed. The teenage years are characterised by intense and volatile emotions and swings of mood. Teenage girls can be very uncertain and unstable.

For the teenager there are lots of unanswered questions. Problems associated with confusion of identity arise as she asks: Who am I? What am I?

A survey by a teen magazine found that 76% of 13-19 year olds reported that pressure from school work and their environment caused their depression. 54% mentioned difficulties in boyfriend-girlfriend relationships and 44% said family conflicts were a source of depression.

The teenage years are confusing ones. Gail Sheehy popularized adult developmental psychology in her book ***Passages***. Sheehy described themes that predominate in ten-year chunks of lives. For the teenager, the passage which needs negotiation is a mere six-year time span. Some would argue that it's the most troubled passage to negotiate. One popular theory suggests that teenagers today are exposed to more stressors than ever before. However, the teenage years have always been troubling times. As early as 1924, Winifred Holtby wrote in ***The Crowded Street***, about her heroine Muriel:

'Being grown-up was puzzling. It seemed to make no difference at all in most things, and then to matter frightfully in quite unexpected ways. It meant, for instance, not so much the assumption of new duties as the acceptance of new values.

Was she more stupid than other people, or did everyone feel like this at first? She was traveling in a land of which she only imperfectly understood the language.'

Negotiating all these changes – the transition from childhood to adulthood, can be fraught with difficulties. It may not take much to tip the balance from being a 'normal' confused teenager in search of her identity to feeling intensely depressed and suicidal.

Shaylee, for instance, had crossed the boundary from 'normal' to troubled. It's a boundary that's easily crossed. Shaylee, did not run away, she decided to stay at home and the whole family went to family therapy. Shaylee's depression had become a family problem. Depression often has this ripple effect on the entire family.

And in Shaylee's case, her family were supportive. They wanted to understand her distress – and they wanted to help.

A DEPRESSIVE PASSAGE

Doubts and uncertainties mark the adolescent identity crisis. Being a teenager means you'll experience maximum uncertainty about who you are and where you are going. But not all teenagers become depressed. Some of them negotiate the teenage years successfully.

Often the teenager's depression is missed or misdiagnosed. In the teenage years, depression tends to wear a different face. School work may fall off and a previously energetic teenager may become fatigued and quiet. She might complain about noises in her ears, dizziness, numbness and tingling in her fingers. The two eating disorders of anorexia and bulimia, stem from poor self-image and a sense of hopelessness and loss of control. Overeating also reflects the teenager's unhappiness. Shoplifting, anti-social behaviour and running away from home are other ways teenagers can act out their depression.

A teenager with poor self-image, and a depression masked by feelings of angry rebellion may turn to the whispered promise of a high through drugs and alcohol. These 'feel good' substances offer respite from low feelings maybe for an hour or so. That promise is enticing. But many of these self-medications – these drugs – are actual depressants and may cause the teenager to go into an even deeper depression.

Kathleen McCoy in her book, **Coping with Teenage Depression**, says:

'Mental health professionals who treat teenagers indicate that most adolescent depression is of the reactive variety. The major challenge, then, is to help the young person discover, explore and work through feelings about the losses and life stresses that have brought about his or her depression.'

She quotes psychiatric sources who claim that manic-depression or bi-polar disorder and chronic depression is not frequent in young people.

Nevertheless, teenagers do suffer depression in large numbers. Alarming figures estimate that the number of high school students who suffer depression ranges from one in five to one in eleven. More disturbingly, in the United States, 5,000 teenagers commit suicide annually. What's more, for every suicide, 50 to 220 teenagers attempt suicide. In fact, suicide is the second leading cause of death in the United States for young people between the ages of 15 and 19. Youth suicide is one of the major social problems facing Australia today. In 1996, there were 84 young female suicides (between the ages of 15 and 24). While young men have a higher suicide rate, young women are 35 times more likely to be admitted to hospital for self-inflicted harm.

THE IMPACT OF BIOLOGY

During the teenage years, girls begin to be much more likely to report depression than boys. The girls who are depressed, report more health problems, more school difficulties and poorer interpersonal and family relationships.

Increase in production of ovarian hormones in girls at puberty does not directly account for increases in rates of depression. Girls do show somewhat elevated levels of depression during the initial activation of the endocrine system, but levels of depression decline once hormonal production becomes stable. Because not every teenage girl becomes depressed, it is important to look at other factors that might cause the depression.

There are substantial individual differences in how girls deal with potentially depression-producing events in their lives. Those girls who can't find a satisfactory and stable self-concept are more vulnerable to depression.

Vulnerability is hard to define. Yet it has something to do with how 'psychologically hardy' a young girl is, how confident she feels in herself, her level of self-esteem and what her support network is like. If she has people around her who care for her, nurture her sense of self and positively reinforce her struggles with dilemmas and decisions then she is likely to be less vulnerable than the young girl who has nagging doubts about her abilities, has a low opinion of herself and has few people around her to encourage and support her thoughts, behaviour and emerging need to be independent.

Even for the well-adjusted adolescent girl, simple problems can take on enormous proportions. A sensitive girl who develops too quickly and leaves behind her girlish body shape and is prone to acne can experience a period of depression. One young client told me that she was extremely embarrassed when she developed a mild case of acne. She felt that it detracted from her overall physical appearance. She sought treatment from a dermatologist, but while she was anxious about her blemishes, she shunned the world as much as she could.

On weekends, she had little social contact and she became increasingly withdrawn and insecure. Her mother was supportive of her and encouraged her to feel good about herself, but it wasn't until her skin had cleared up that she felt less depressed about her image. She told me that she needed a lot of 'false confidence' to re-enter her social world – and that her experience of depression and withdrawal from social life had strengthened her. In her words, she claimed to *'really understand how awful it is – and how depressed you can get – when you have some physical problem.'*

In fact, many teenagers experience depression because they 'feel different' from their peers. The young girl who at 15 looks several years younger may get depressed wondering if she'll ever grow up. Similarly, a young girl who has to wear a corrective brace for scoliosis may feel very different from her friends. A young epileptic girl whom I saw said she felt different 'all the time' and this occasionally depressed her. Yet another teenage girl confessed that she felt depressed 'most of the time' because the strict regimen of her diabetic medical condition set her apart from her peers.

These teenage girls who feel different and get depressed can be helped by allowing them to discover and understand what they can do, rather than what they cannot. Tania, a teenager who has lived with diabetes most of her life – and struggled with depression said: *I've learned to not make my diabetes the central focus of my life. It's only a small part of who I am – I'm a strong and enthusiastic person – I'm learning to love life – I just happen to have diabetes.'*

It may be helpful to point out that other people, some of them well-known celebrities can lead a full and productive life and live with their medical condition. Such role models for teenagers with disabilities are important. They encourage these young people to look up to others who cope with disability and chronic illness and are productive and content.

The mind-body connection cannot be underestimated. Teenagers who are comfortable with themselves and their bodies – their strengths and their weaknesses are more likely to cope with stress and less inclined to become depressed.

THE GIRL WHO CUT HERSELF

Like Lady Diana, Miranda, aged 15, slashed her arms and legs. When she came to see me for counselling, she said she felt *'stressed – you know really tense – and depressed, feeling no good about myself.'.*

When I met Miranda, she was wearing slacks and a long-sleeved shirt. It is well known that women who harm themselves go to great lengths to hide their scars. There is a great deal of shame associated with the act of self-mutilation.

However, when the young woman harms herself she sees this as her only option. Her low self-esteem, her hatred for her body and her sense of desperation leads her to disperse her tension, allowing her body to deal with unbearable emotion.

Miranda told me she injured herself in private to release the 'badness' she felt. She spoke about her psychological distress:

'I felt so bad. Down, lonely, tense, agitated – all these emotions rolled into one – feeling bad. It was like I felt this pressure building up inside me and that only cutting myself would relieve it. I remember the first time it happened. I was lying in the bath trying to remain calm as my parents argued downstairs. Somehow I felt responsible for their arguing. I thought I was bad. I'd been feeling really low for a few months – I couldn't talk to my mom anymore. We'd been really good friends – then I don't know – things between us got difficult. Anyway, there I was, in the bath, putting my head under water to block out the sounds. Then it suddenly occurred to me – why not use the razorblade I shave my legs with to cut myself? I took it, and then sank the blade into my arm. It felt good – like popping a balloon, like purging. I just watched the blood feather out into the bath water – and I felt much calmer, much better.'

Miranda's words tell us the agony she felt as the 'bad' girl responsible for her parents arguing – and then the ecstasy she felt when she 'let out' her badness. Cutting herself felt good – for the moment. But in the long-term, self-destructive behaviour is likely to reinforce the depression Miranda felt in the first place.

There are no reliable statistics on how many women self-mutilate. These women rarely end up in emergency departments. However, it is known that it's far more likely to involve women than men. These women are usually aged between 15 and 30, and although some women in their thirties and forties continue to injure themselves, it is rarer in the fifties plus group.

Women who harm themselves are usually depressed, sometimes angry, although they may not recognise this, and feeling under a lot of pressure. What these women say, time and again, is that when the knife goes in, there's a tremendous release of tension. One woman put it this way: *'Cutting myself gives me the control I haven't got and it's a way of venting my anger. In a way, it's therapeutic.'*

Such an expression of inner pain signals a distress and helplessness which can be addressed better by allowing the woman to articulate her pain, her anger and her sense of hopelessness. Having someone to talk to, to be able to let out the pain in words, rather than self-harming actions, is crucial. Unlike Lady Diana, some women don't feel they can tell anyone. They feel ashamed and guilty – and they're worried that others might judge them harshly. As Lady Diana implied in her interview with Martin Bashir, having someone listen to you, having someone take you seriously might make all the difference.

Making the difference can be achieved if our basic needs are met – rather than denied. Understanding basic needs is crucial – for both the teenage girl and her parents.

HELP LINE: THREE BASIC HUMAN NEEDS

The three basic needs of human beings are: love, understanding, choice.

When we feel loved and loving, we feel:
warmth, belonging, happy, closeness, affectionate

When we feel unloved, we feel:
sad, rejected, lost, pain, emptiness, fear

When we understand and are understood, we feel:
accepted, safe, relaxed, self-esteem, valued

When we do not understand, and believe people don't understand us, we feel:
anxious, panicky, lost, isolated, that life is meaningless

When we feel that we can make choices and that we are in control of our lives, we feel:
satisfaction, energetic, motivated, powerful, strong

When we seem to have no choices, we feel:
anger, depression, helpless, resigned

Feeling loved, understood and believing we have choices in life are important for everyone – it defines our humaness. For the teenager, whose life often seems chaotic and out of control, feeling loved, understood and being allowed to make choices and life decisions, are important and empowering ingredients in their lives.

As a parent, it might be tempting to make judgements about your teenager's behaviour. It also might be tempting to do things for her, rather than letting her discover and learn through life experience. Often parents will want to 'protect' their daughters from possible harsh consequences, however, the truth is, that a lesson lived is a lesson learned. However much you might want to spare your daughter, it's unfair to take over – she has the right to her emerging adult status, and with it, the responsibility to make choices and decisions. If a parent is seen to 'take over' too vigorously – however well-intentioned their motives – the teenage girl will begin to resent what she considers 'interference'.

TEENAGERS AND DRUG USE

A 1999 study found that young women start using Ecstasy or MDMA at age 17 compared with 18 for young men. Also, it seems that Ecstasy is the only illicit drug used more widely by women than men.

Drug use is a very difficult problem to face. Often parents are disinclined to believe their teenagers are experimenting with drugs. Many parents suspect drug abuse, but ignore it, hoping that their suspicions are unfounded and that the situation will simply improve. Sitting down with teenage girls and confronting them about drug use can be self-defeating. A sense of confusion and betrayal may result – for both teenagers and their parents.

THE GIRL WHO RAN AWAY

As I listen to Stephanie, I'm reminded of the girl who keeps a diary in **Go Ask Alice**, the diary of a young drug dependent girl who runs away and becomes a 'baby prostitute'. Although she returns home, her drug dependency escalates and she eventually overdoses. The diarist reveals to us her struggles with adolescence, peer relationships, school, and parents – particularly her father. She finds temporary escape in drugs and running away from home. Only every time she comes down from her drug high, or returns home, her life seems unchanged. Each time, she believes that drugs will offer her a permanent solution to life's problems. She writes in her diary:

> 'Then I talked to Alice, who I met just sitting stoned on the curb. She didn't know whether she was running away from something or running to something, but she admitted that deep in her heart she wanted to go home.
>
> The others I talked to, the ones who had homes, all seemed to want to go back, but felt they couldn't because that would mean giving up their identity. It made me think about the hundreds of thousands of kids who have run away and are wandering around all over the place. Where do they come from? Where do they even manage to crash for the night? Most of them don't have any money and don't have anywhere to go.
>
> I think I'll go into child guidance when I get out of school. Or maybe I should become a psychologist. At least I'd be able to understand where kids are at and maybe that would help compensate for what I've done to my family and myself. Perhaps it was even right for me to go through all this suffering so that I could be more understanding and tolerant of the rest of humanity.
>
> Oh dear wonderful, trusting, friendly Diary, that's exactly what I'll do. I'll spend the rest of my life helping people who are just like me! I feel so good and happy. I finally have something to do for the rest of my life. Wow! I'm through with drugs too. I've used the hard stuff only a few times and I don't like it. I don't like any of it. The uppers or downers, I'm through with the whole mess. Absolutely and completely and forever, really I am.'

The diarist didn't give up drugs, and within three weeks of resolving not to keep another diary she was dead.

Getting high and running away in the hope of leaving your worries behind – or to have them magically disappear on your return – are escapist thinking and behaviours. They are not grounded in reality – and the teenager is not reality-testing her expectations and subsequent behaviours.

Stephanie had run away from home too. She, like Alice, had become involved in the drug scene. However, she went to a girls' detention centre and met a counsellor who changed her life. In fact, she also met an older girl, who had a history of drug use and detention, and Stephanie had learned a lot about the downside of independence – and rebellion. With a lot of support and a large dose of motivation, Stephanie was able to turn her life around. She and her family came to see me for family therapy, recognising that if one member of the family has a problem – they all have a problem.

In **Go Ask Alice**, a psychologist, James Hemming gives his comments. These comments reflect issues involved in both Alice's internal and external worlds. Her lack of self-esteem and her attraction to risk-taking behaviours were combined with parental and societal expectations of who she should be – and this proved to be a powerful magnet to a scene which promised good feelings and an unconditional acceptance. As James Hemming said: *'Drugs got their grip on Alice because they made her feel 'wonderful', whereas she usually felt inferior and unwanted.'*

Stephanie told me she felt that her parents often didn't listen to her. And their expectations of her future were too high. She felt a lot of pressure to be 'the good daughter and do them proud'. She said,

> *'The real problem was the feelings I had. I thought that no-one had problems like me. I felt misunderstood. Drugs made me feel good. I remember after a friend injected me for the first time, all my feelings were removed from me. All the bad things were blocked out. I thought I'd found the answer.'*

But Stephanie hadn't found the answer. Months after her first shot of heroin, all she had were questions. Questions about how she had betrayed herself and her parents, and how she had allowed herself to sink so low.

Her parents were motivated to help her. Looking back, they could see how things had gone wrong. They believed they were protecting Stephanie, wanting the best for her – without checking out with Stephanie what she wanted to do with her life.

KEEPING LINES OF COMMUNICATION OPEN

Talking and listening are important with teenage children – for both parents and teenagers. So often, teenagers become depressed because they believe no-one cares, they feel misunderstood and alienated even from parents who are caring and concerned. Keeping lines of communication open between the teenager and her parents is a challenging task – but ultimately, a most rewarding one. As Stephanie said, she believed her parents 'didn't listen to her'. Being heard, when you're a teenager and your life is topsy-turvy, is crucial for your mental health and sense of well-being in the world.

What is good listening? Listening is an active process of receiving, processing and interpreting information. It means more than just being present. For instance, you can be present at a play or a concert and pay no attention to it. Being present means being involved – paying attention, understanding and evaluating. Effective listening also requires your alertness. You have to be able to pick up cues. Sometimes these are non-verbal – so watch carefully. Listening also means checking out that you heard the message as it was intended – and offering feedback as it is needed. To truly be an effective listener, you have to let the teenager know that you have heard and that you understand and you have an opinion on the matter.

LISTEN EMPATHICALLY

When we listen empathically, we listen from the point of view of the speaker, rather than from our own. We put ourselves in their place and attempt to see the world from their perspective. By listening empathically, you respond to the speaker's needs rather than your own. It's also a good idea to reflect back to the speaker your sense of her feelings. For instance:

- reflect back your understanding of her feelings, 'You sound really angry about that' or 'You seem to be anxious about performing in the school band'
- give your teenager permission to express her feelings by talking about how difficult it is to express feelings, for example, 'It's really difficult to express feelings at a time like this,' or 'You must feel really hurt by that'
- avoid judgemental responses, for example, 'Cheer up, things will get better', or 'Don't feel so bad, in time you'll forget about it'
- use reinforcing comments to let your teenager know that you understand what she's saying and encourage her to continue talking. You can use comments like. 'I understand', or 'Right' or 'I get it', or 'I see'

E. M. Forster once said: *'Only connect!'*

The following checklist begins this process of connection for you and your teenage daughter.

CHECKLIST: LEARNING TO CONNECT – SOME CONSIDERATIONS

1. Emotional responsiveness

How emotionally responsive are you to each other? Warmth and caring – and a flexible attitude need to be openly given and received. Parents and daughters need to be sufficiently in touch with themselves – and feel safe – to express a range of thoughts and feelings to each other. It is most important to be genuine and sincere in your expression of feelings.

2. Respect

How respectful are you towards each other? Respect means allowing the other person – your daughter – to grow as a separate human being. You are able to help – and take pleasure in her unfolding. Being possessive and controlling are the antithesis of respect. You must understand that respecting another person means that you are secure enough in yourself to allow that person the psychological space to be herself.

3. Considerateness and caring

Are you thoughtful about another person's feelings?
Considerateness involves being aware of another person's needs. By being considerate, you can show your teenager that you care.

4. Sense of humour

Does the child in your teenager appeal to the child in you? By learning to laugh and appreciate each other's sense of humour, you can enhance the good times you have together and ease the tense times in your relationship.

5. Trustworthiness and commitment

Can you depend on each other? Your relationship involves contracts – both implicit and explicit. These contracts or agreements relate to matters such as not violating family rules, being home on time, keeping promises and generally acting in a reliable and dependable manner. A committed person does not breach trust.

6. Compatibility of values

Do you share the underlying principles and priorities on which you base your life? Although differences in values are inevitable, you need to feel compatible with each other's major values in order to sustain a respectful relationship.

These considerations are a good beginning point. Parents can share their thoughts and feelings with their teenage daughters on such considerations. A teenage girl can begin to risk letting her parents know where she stands. By beginning to understand each other's point of view, more realistic expectations can be reached. Then – be prepared to compromise!

CIRCLE THIS

Teenagers want and need a world that is separate from their parents. Give your teenage girl the space and time to be reflective – that will mean a better transition to adulthood.

WHAT YOU CAN DO IF YOUR TEENAGER IS DEPRESSED

Empathise with your teenage girl. Listen actively to her concerns – and don't dismiss her perspective as trivial.

Even if your teenage daughter is driving you mad with her depression and general 'moping' or risk-taking behaviour, let her know that her behaviour is affecting you. Parents are not perfect. Neither should they pretend to be. Letting your teenage daughter see your vulnerability will help facilitate her own feelings to come to the surface. Let your daughter know you, as a parent who is caring – and human. Sharing vulnerability can be the beginning of a new and better communication pattern. By sharing vulnerability, you are giving your teenage daughter the permission to find her way out of her depression – by allowing her to express her innermost fears and darkest doubts about herself and her place in the world.

CIRCLE THIS

Sometimes your teenage girl just won't talk – no matter how available you are. Respect her reticence and her wishes. Show her you respect her and she will feel valued. Gently remind her that you are there for her and interested in what she has to say.

Read the following whimsical comment on the value of listening – and learn to listen carefully to your teenager.

Listen

When I ask you to listen to me
and you start giving advice
you have not done what I asked.

When I ask you to listen to me
and you begin to tell me why I shouldn't feel that way,
you are trampling on my feelings

When I ask you to listen to me
and you feel you have to do something to solve my problems,
you have failed me, strange as that may seem.

Listen! All I ask is that you listen.
Not talk or do – just hear me.
Advice is cheap
and available every day in the newspaper

And I can DO for myself; I am not helpless.
Maybe discouraged and faltering, but not helpless.

When you do something for me that I can and need to do for myself,
you contribute to my fear and weakness.

But when you accept as a simple fact that I do feel what I feel, no matter how irrational,
then I quit trying to convince you and can get about the business of understanding what's behind this irrational feeling.
And when that's clear, the answers are obvious and
I don't need advice.

So please listen and just hear me, and if you want
to talk, wait a minute for your turn;
and I'll listen to you.

Anonymous

6

BIRTH BLUES

'I wish someone had said:
'The baby's fine, but how are you?''

MARNI, 32

Marni laughs as she recalls how excited she was when her doctor confirmed she was pregnant. She faxed her mother the simple message: 'Get knitting', and left a voicemail for her husband saying, 'Test positive – dinner and champagne at 7.00'.

Marni is the sort of competent, sensible and in her words, 'practical' woman whom you expect to be able to cope well in any situation. As she speaks, however, I get the impression that she still is amazed that she hadn't breezed through pregnancy and childbirth without a hiccup. She had a healthy, uncomplicated pregnancy and an easy birth. But four days after her son was born, she became teary, anxious and had pronounced mood swings. Marni was unaccustomed to being so emotionally vulnerable. Marni experienced the 'baby blues' after the birth of her first child – a much wanted and planned baby. Marni's vulnerability to depression is much more common than most people know.

THE 'BABY BLUES' –
A COMMON OCCURRENCE

Giving birth has long been associated with mood change. In fact, in the days immediately following birth, between two-thirds and three-quarters of women experience what's called the 'baby blues'. These baby blues usually affect women between three to five days after they give birth. Some women have called this time the 'ten day weepies' which refers to how long they experience the emotional upheaval. In fact, in the nineteenth century it was known as 'milk fever', as it coincided with those days when milk appeared in quantity in the woman's breasts. Women who have experienced the baby blues say they alternate between highs and lows – feeling very happy one moment and low and distressed another. They feel weepy and their crying can be triggered by little upsets and even by sheer happiness.

AN INTERESTING FINDING

Dr Irvin D. Yalom led a team of four psychiatrists who studied a group of 39 women before delivery and for the first 10 days after birth. They found that two-thirds of the women had crying episodes lasting at least five minutes during the 10 days after birth, and five of these women cried continuously for more than two hours. After the first eight days there was a reduction in their crying. When the team compared this with the 10 days studied during pregnancy, they found that the women's crying episodes were three times higher after delivery than during their pregnancy. Another finding was that during their pregnancy, the women's tears rarely lasted longer than five minutes.

They also found that often the women didn't cry from sadness, but for a number of other reasons such as, reading the birth announcement, when they received too little or too much attention from the nurses, if they had insufficient milk and relief that labour was over.

Marni's baby blues were not as pronounced as some women's can be. Marni says she knows of one woman who spent the first two weeks bursting into tears over the smallest things – at the sight of flowers, her husband telling her of his promotion, being told her baby was beautiful and receiving baby clothes from friends and family.

Women who experience the baby blues often say they feel out of control and 'silly'. They see their teariness as a sign of weakness, of not being able to cope. Yet, it is a common experience – and no woman should feel ashamed.

> **CIRCLE THIS**
>
> Women and their partners need to be warned during antenatal classes of the possibility of some form of maternal depression occurring. The public should be better educated and women should be given permission to seek out the help they need if they find themselves acting in unexpected ways and feeling at the end of their tether. We all have the responsibility of being more aware of the unexpected torment that can lead to frustration, desperation, and occasionally tragedy.

Marni was fortunate that her symptoms of crying for no apparent reason, having trouble sleeping, lacking concentration and suffering anxiety attacks settled down after eight days. But her comment, *'I wish someone had said, 'the baby's fine, but how are you?'* captures her feeling of being neglected. Everyone, it seemed to her, was concerned for the baby and no-one asked her how she felt.

There are other women, who are not so fortunate. For them, depression after delivery, is more serious.

MATERNAL BLISS AND POST-NATAL DEPRESSION

This more serious depression is called post-natal or postpartum depression and it is still shrouded by as many myths as motherhood is itself. It usually begins two to six weeks after childbirth, and it can last for months or years. The image of mother and child bonding and the maternal bliss the woman feels as she adopts her new role is sometimes blurred by her intense feelings of depression.

Diandra, 31, a first-time mum did not experience the maternal bliss she had expected. She said she missed out on the 'happy mum' syndrome:

No-one tells you it won't be like you daydreamed it would be. You know, everything being beautiful – the idea of the smiling Madonna and beautiful child. I had a huge feeling of being let down – you know, like I'd been betrayed. I hadn't been warned how awful it could be. I absolutely thrived

during my pregnancy – I was healthy and vibrant – I even grew to love my increasingly awkward shape.
'But about three weeks after my son was born I became helpless, miserable and depressed. Instead of enjoying him, of being happy, I was miserable and feeling like a freak. If only someone had warned me that I might suffer these miseries and that it's kinda normal, I wouldn't have felt so bad.'

It can be very distressing for women who have been vital during their pregnancy and awaiting the birth of their baby with joy, to find that they feel negative, flat and depressed. A sense of guilt and shame can overcome such a woman. Sometimes, women may not recognise their depression. They might feel utter exhaustion, a lower quality of life and a feeling of irritability, yet not know they are post-natally depressed. Some women begin to wonder about their moral fibre and self-control and begin to feel guilty about their temper and tears.

According to Dr Wohlreich, of Pennsylvania Hospital's Postpartum Disorders Project:

'Postpartum depression is highly treatable through short-term psychotherapy, medication, and other supportive measures. Many mothers who receive treatment recover within weeks.'

More often called post-natal depression, it affects up to 30% of women. Women usually report having difficulty eating and sleeping, endless exhaustion, an inability to cope, loss of self-esteem and feelings of despair.

It is important that a woman who experiences these sorts of symptoms gets the help she needs – and deserves. As one psychologist said:
'People – both lay and professional can have difficulty understanding post-natal depression. It needs more understanding by everybody. We need to educate everyone.'

Clarissa, 25, experienced a post-natal depression after the birth of her first child. She describes how she had trouble coping, how she wandered around in a foggy state, spending more time in bed than she thought she should. Her only salvation was a very understanding husband. She said:

'I felt like such a rotten person, wife and mother. I felt lonely and isolated. The only thing that kept me going was I knew that Pete would be home at quarter past six – he was so nice. He came home and did almost everything I couldn't face during the day. I felt terribly guilty and inadequate. But I also had these scary feelings – I wanted to be a baby. I didn't want to have to care for a baby – I wanted to become one. I resented my baby – and that really scared me. My therapist told me this is called regression – I wanted time to go backwards. I felt better after she told me I wasn't the only one who had these crazy feelings.'

The explanation Clarissa had been given by her therapist relates to the idea that to a woman robbed of her coping resources and feeling depressed, a baby can seem like a demanding and draining little creature who wants all her attention. Just when the mother could be experiencing great happiness, she feels miserable and helpless.

Linden, 28 experienced a post-natal depression after the birth of her second child. She had not experienced depression after her first baby, although she did have a few 'weepy' days. She said:

'It's really hard to pinpoint when I got depressed. It must have been about a month after Gemma was born. I felt so many different ways – often within the space of a couple of hours. At times I felt nothing. At other times I felt down in the pits. Everything seemed to crowd in around me. I felt I had to be the perfect mother – which I hadn't felt so strongly when Robbie was born.

'I felt like I was in a maze – everything seemed to overwhelm me. I had real trouble coping. I can remember walking around in a dazed state. Sometimes I couldn't believe all this was happening to me. At first when I spoke to my doctor about it, he wasn't concerned, but a few weeks later, he took one look at me and prescribed anti-depressants. I also went into counselling – my husband insisted on it. Now that it's behind me, I find it all too distressing to think about. But do you know what? I'm a little scared that if I have another baby the same thing might happen again.'

Linden is not alone in her fear that she might experience another post-natal depression. Some women put off another pregnancy for years fearing the worst. Yet the evidence is not strong that once a woman has experienced a post-natal depression she has a greater chance of doing so again. However, the woman's memory of the intensity of the depression may be so overwhelming that she convinces herself that she will experience the same misery again.

This happened to 30 year old Laraine. She is an example of a woman who desperately wanted a baby. An early miscarriage meant that Laraine was even more intent on having a second healthy and uneventful pregnancy. Having children was very important to her. When she married, she told her husband she wanted at least four children. Laraine's post-natal depression came as a complete shock. Since childhood, when she'd discovered she had been adopted, Laraine had wanted children of her own. But her post-natal depression had made her re-think her ambitions of a large family. She said:

'I wanted to have children so desperately. I knew I had to have children – my own flesh and blood – and I wanted to raise them myself – not like my birth mother had done. Then I had the miscarriage and I was devastated. When I became pregnant again, I felt so positive, and I knew everything would be alright. But then, a few weeks after my daughter was born, I became very depressed. I loved her so much, but I resented the responsibility.

'I suddenly felt overwhelmed – I can recall almost everything overwhelmed me. I couldn't decide the simplest thing – making decisions was impossible for me. And then I began to worry. I spent hours worrying about whether my baby daughter was sleeping well enough, feeding enough – I even worried if the formula was too hot or too cold. I felt so alone. I didn't know of any other mothers who felt like me. And here I was – with a really wanted baby – and feeling so lousy.

'The depression didn't lift until she was about 14 months old, when she made fewer demands – and I didn't feel so responsible. That whole depression experience has made me wonder whether I want another child. I was so enthusiastic and ready, but being a mother was different from what I expected. Now I wonder whether I can go through it all again.'

Laraine's story shows us that even a woman who is positive about her pregnancy and happy during it, is not necessarily spared of post-natal depression. There is no contradiction between a woman being seemingly ready for motherhood and the reality of becoming a mother, which might bring with it, anxieties and fears – and a sense of not being able to cope. Some women find that they feel confused and helpless. They feel lost – and a sense of loss.

FEELING LOST AND A SENSE OF LOSS

Clarissa also spoke of this loss. She believed she and her husband had lost many of the good things in their relationship – walks in the park, visits to galleries and museums, going out to dinner. But, it was her jealousy of her baby that brought this sense of loss into sharp focus. She was jealous of her child. She said: *'When my husband cuddled the baby, I felt left out, neglected. I felt like I'd lost out to my baby – she was taking my place in my husband's affections.'*

Linden also referred to this sense of loss when she said: *'I seemed to have gone from complete freedom to having to rely on others – calling babysitters each time we wanted to go out, that sort of thing. It was a big adjustment to make.'*

It's easy to see how the arrival of a new baby can lead to a feeling of loss: a loss of independence, loss of relative freedoms, loss of social contacts, loss of status, loss of earnings – and perhaps even a perceived loss of an exclusive relationship with a husband or partner. These losses may or may not be compensated for by the birth of the baby.

The vulnerability of the baby may make the mother feel anxious and the constant demands can lead to a sense of fragmentation. And a sense of submerged identity. Many women report having difficulty focusing on tasks and as one woman put it, *'I sort of felt lost at sea.'*

A popular British television personality, Esther Rantzen, spoke of her post-natal depression and the losses she felt:

'Yes, I'm lucky. A great job, a loving husband, nanny to look after the baby... but I was utterly defenceless when it happened to me. For a month it was utter hell. I felt as if I was going insane. I have heard myself shouting at my husband in an unforgiveable way and yelling that I must see a doctor, that I was going

mad. There were awful attacks of shaking, stumbling, and trembling. I suffered from what I call 'mind slip'. I couldn't concentrate. I could not even dictate letters because I was getting my words mixed up. It was as if I'd lost a part of myself.'

This sense of loss that Esther Rantzen articulates is a common theme among women who experience post-natal depression. According to Dr Marie-Paule Austin, a psychiatrist, *'Society idealises motherhood. Everybody's meant to be happy and content but often that's not true. A child radically changes the dynamics of relationships, you get little sleep, have little time and the child always has to take priority. For career women, particularly, this is hard to adjust to.'*

A woman might be thrilled and delighted to have a baby, yet at the same time be overwhelmed by strong feelings brought about by the demand of the dependent, helpless bundle that is her baby. She might feel she's lost out – and feel trapped, angry, depressed and guilty. Sometimes the experience of having the baby is not what she imagined or hoped for. There may be a gap between her fantasy baby and her real baby. The baby may not be as pretty as she'd hoped for, or she may have a boy instead of a hoped-for girl, she may feel a failure because she didn't have a natural birth or she can't breastfeed, or the baby that was intended to mend the marriage has caused further rifts.

Too often, the fairytale picture of the perfect mother and the happy baby are presented in the media. What Diandra called 'the happy mum' syndrome has wide currency. Although women attend ante-natal classes, very rarely is the downside of early motherhood mentioned. Esther German, a clinical psychologist who works with women comments, *'It's taboo to discuss even the most normal reactions to motherhood that don't fit the picture, and often, it's mothers who don't want to know. I go to prenatal classes to tell people about PND (post-natal depression) and sometimes they'll react as though it's contagious to even talk about it.'* Perhaps this reaction is based partly on fear – and superstition that by discussing what might go wrong, you can jinx yourself. In part, it is probably a defence mechanism like denial as well. Denial that the woman might not be able to cope – and a fear that if she can't she must be a 'bad mother'.

In a powerful telemovie, ***Do I have to kill my child?***, a young mother attempts to draw attention to her inability to cope. She feels lethargic and depressed and resents her new-born child. No-one takes her calls for help seriously. Everyone listens, but no-one hears – they all believe she really can cope. In one scene, she tells a kindly older neighbour 'You know, it's a terrible thing to say, but sometimes I think I could kill him'. Her neighbour's response is, 'We all feel that way sometimes honey.' The young mother's frustration escalates until her desperation is acted out by harming her child.

Surely now, someone will take her seriously.

Post-natal depression can be experienced as mild, moderate or severe. Factors which may contribute to its onset and continuation include difficulties with the baby, relationship problems, difficulty sleeping, trouble in breastfeeding and the demands of other small children.

THE WORKINGS OF A FRENZIED MIND – 'I WASN'T IN THE SAME WORLD'

A third more extreme form of maternal depression is puerperal psychosis. A woman suffering from this form of depression has delusions, hallucinations, and may threaten to take her own life or injure the baby. This is a much rarer form of depression than either the 'baby blues' or post-natal depression. The majority of women who experience this depression show manic-depressive qualities. Unfortunately, it is this more extreme form of depression that makes the headlines in the form of horrifying tales of tragedy. Examples of headlines include: 'New mother jumps to her death', 'Wife stabs her husband', 'Mother drowns baby girl', and 'Mother kills her three children.'

Hospitalisation is essential for most women who experience this form of depression – and lose touch with reality. This depression can develop quickly bringing with it a complete change of personality overnight. Many women become depressed after labor.

Samantha experienced a complete change in herself after she gave birth. She said:

'I wasn't in the same world. The day after the Caesarean I woke up and found the world looked different. It smelt different – and I thought my food smelled – maybe the hospital staff was trying to poison me. I felt like I was being sucked into a deep vacuum at great speed.'

These can be frightening feelings and sensations and according to Samantha, it was only speedy hospitalisation and treatment with anti-depressants and ECT (electo-convulsive therapy) that saved her. Electro-convulsive therapy or ECT, or as it is more popularly known, 'shock treatment' has developed a controversial and fearsome reputation. ECT has been used for over 50 years. Today the procedure is much improved, although there are some undesirable effects, such as confusion, headaches and temporary memory loss. Studies show that ECT seems to be as effective as anti-depressant medication on hospitalised patients. It has also been suggested that for people with severe depression, who are unresponsive to medication and therapy, ECT is an option to consider.

Often the delusions the woman has centre on the baby. For instance, a woman may believe her baby is deformed, or the incarnation of evil and because of these delusions she may try to harm either the baby or herself or both. Women who develop this form of psychosis – and lose touch with reality – sometimes show early signs of distress. They might seem over-active, suspicious, tense, anxious, complaining, overdemanding and often have difficulty sleeping.

Puerperal psychosis is a serious condition, and women who experience it are confused and muddled in their thinking. Often they have very bizarre thoughts. For instance, one woman was later told she had been hammering her baby's head, with seeming lack of concern for the baby's welfare. Apparently she had said, 'It's not the right shape. It's too long – I have to make it the right shape.' Another woman had confessed to wanting to stick a pin in her baby's pupils because his big blue eyes had disturbed her too much. She found her baby son's stare too penetrating. She believed he was trying to hypnotize her.

A confusion of senses occurs in this sort of depression. Seeing and hearing people who are not there as well as tasting and smelling things which are not present can be a frightening and traumatic experience for all concerned. A husband or partner might be challenged to deal with such irrational behaviour. Support and understanding – and a large measure of patience – are required for all family members. A woman who experiences puerperal psychosis is at the mercy of forces beyond her control and cannot be told to pull herself together.

For these women, who are so removed from reality, and whose irrational acts are disturbing, prompt medical treatment is essential. Very often these women have very little memory of their disturbance – or at least the more extreme aspects of it. This might well be nature's way of being kind to the woman. Sometimes, women like Samantha can remember parts of what had happened and feel guilty. They are unable to comprehend how it was possible for them to have behaved as they did.

FACT FILE

There are three distinct conditions which fall under the general heading 'birth blues':

1. Baby blues
– an estimated 60% to 80% of women might experience this
– time-limited, usually around 10 days

2. Post-natal depression
– affects between 10% – 30% of mothers
– usually appears within six weeks of the birth

3. Puerperal psychosis
– incidence is rare, between 1 to 2 per 1,000 births
– characterised by delusions, irrational behaviour and hallucinations
– prompt treatment is essential

In the area of post-natal depression, there are many myths. It helps if a woman has some knowledge so that she is in a position to challenge myths. Myths can create unnecessary anxiety. Look at the following myths and the facts which challenge them:

A difficult pregnancy means the woman will experience post-natal depression.
There is no evidence that a troublesome pregnancy forecasts trouble ahead. By the same token, a trouble-free pregnancy does not guarantee total post-natal tranquility.

A lengthy and difficult labor leads to post-natal depression.
There is no known correlation between the type and length of labour and post-natal depression. However, anxiety before and during labour can mean a lengthy labour.

Post-natal depression only occurs in natural mothers.
Studies show that post-natal depression may occur in an adoptive mother. This finding lends weight to the idea that there are psychological and emotional causes, along with any hormonal factors.

Only women experience post-natal depression.
Some twenty years ago, Dr G. Zelboorg and Dr W. Wainwright found that some fathers also develop a depression, occasionally serious enough to be treated and hospitalized.

Sexual difficulties are part of the post-natal experience.
Any sexual problems which occur are usually short-lived. There is no evidence that post-natal depression leads to chronic sexual difficulties. However, as mentioned earlier, a demanding partner or fear of another pregnancy, and avoidance of physical discomfort may postpone full sexual activity for a little while.

Now that you have the facts, it's easier to dismiss some of the mythology around post-natal depression. Some of these myths only make you feel anxious and guilty – so discard them!

WHY DO WOMEN GET DEPRESSED POST-NATALLY?

There are competing explanations for a woman's vulnerability to birth blues. First, there's the hormonal explanation. Both oestrogen and progesterone levels are very high during pregnancy then drop dramatically in the first week after the baby is delivered. The hormonal explanation attributes depression to an imbalance in the oestrogen/progesterone ratio, unusually high levels of progesterone or to abnormally rapidly declining levels of progesterone. According to this theory, a woman's depression may relate to her body's regulation of oestrogen and progesterone during pregnancy and immediately after delivery. It is believed that these hormonal upheavals are principally responsible for the 'baby blues', which women experience a few days after delivery.

Secondly, there are social and stress explanations of post-natal depression, which develops some weeks after the birth. If you recall the 'Life Events and Difficulties' questionnaire you'll remember seeing that pregnancy and birth are considered to be events which call for a substantial readjustment in a woman's life. For some women, these events represent overwhelming new challenges. The immense practical demands on the new mother, preparing the baby, fitting in feeds, a baby's incessant crying and the transition to a taxing new life-style may engender a sense of inadequacy in the woman – and depression. Very often women find themselves more socially isolated and isolation can lead to a sense of loneliness, which can be depressing.

Linden, who spoke earlier, found that having two children isolated her more than one. She was ruled by a stricter routine which revolved mainly around her baby daughter, Gemma. She discovered in her counselling sessions that she needed time for herself – and that she should have this time and enjoy this time, without feeling guilty. Her solution was to join a healthclub, where the children could be minded. Then she set herself a demanding four-times-a-week schedule. Within a month, she found she felt refreshed and less stressed. She said,

> 'Going to the gym has revived me. It's given me time for myself and somewhere outside the home where I can go and do something unmum-like. It makes for a break and a good workout leaves me feeling energized and positive – really ready to cope with the kids! Even my husband, who was a bit iffy about my gym activity, has come to see how good it is for me. I've started to dump the guilt as well – because I can see the benefits for everyone.'

This theme of 'time for myself' is one that crops up a lot. So is the guilt. Many mothers are guilt-ridden about doing something for themselves. They seem to be programmed to do everything for everyone else – but leave themselves out. It's important to work on letting go of the idea that to do something for yourself you are being selfish. You deserve to treat yourself well.

Marni also talked about not having time to herself, and the need to develop an attitude that allows you to take time out. She said,

> 'Not having time to myself got me down at first. Then a friend who'd been there and done that, told me how to free myself up – just for some bits of time now and then. I get a sitter in or leave the baby with a friend – and just go out and take a breather from the demands. I think you have to do that otherwise you'd go mad.'

Another recurring theme is the idea that to survive the birth blues, a woman had to have support from people around her.

SUPPORT TO HELP YOU THROUGH

Esther Rantzen who spoke earlier managed to overcome her depression by talking to significant people about it. Confiding in others and getting their support are crucial ingredients in getting over birth blues. Esther Rantzen said:

> 'I was one of the lucky ones, though. I managed to get out of it by talking over my feelings with everyone from my husband, friends, and family, to my health visitor who was wonderful, and a marvelous doctor came round and listened.'

It takes courage often to let another person, however supportive, know how awful you feel. You may believe that others won't understand why you're feeling so low at such a seemingly happy time. You may feel guilty about feeling so blue.

One woman, Jenny, 36 is an advocate of talking things out with trusted people – and recognises the value of support. She said:

> *'My advice to mothers going through post-natal depression would be this: have faith in yourself that you will get through it but seek help, either from a medical person or a friend who you can call at 3.00am and say, 'The child's screaming, I'm going mad, come and take it away.' I'm not saying don't have a baby because there are many rewards and pluses but I do think we need to take this problem very seriously.'*

Confiding in others and knowing that they are available as support to you – to help you through the hard times, both emotionally and physically, is essential if we are to take the 'problem' of post-natal depression 'seriously' as Jenny suggests.

Talking out any concerns you have helps your mental health. It brings back a sense of balance in your life. This helps take you out of that downward spiral mentioned earlier and into a more positive, upward spiral.

Finding the right level of support for you is a first step in helping yourself overcome your birth blues. Another beginning step is to begin organising your life – to set yourself a routine – and introduce some structure into your day.

CIRCLE THIS

Setting yourself a routine in the early days with a new baby brings structure to what sometimes feels like chaos. You'll find that by being disciplined about tasks and activities, you can achieve more and feel better about yourself. Try writing yourself out a timetable for the day – and you might find that it is less effort simply to do something at the time set out on your piece of paper than to find the willpower and impetus to do the task when it demands to be done – and you've put off doing it!

'NOT TONIGHT, DARLING...'

Sometimes women experiencing even a mild form of baby blues have little or no interest in sex. There are good reasons for not having sex for some time, even after an easy birth. A woman's body has to adapt to the tremendous changes in levels of hormones, which are responsible for creating sexual desire. And this adaptation takes time. Massive physical changes take place in the womb and vagina as a result of childbirth. If she has had an episiotomy, she may be tender and anxious about having sex.

Regaining sensitivity and having pleasurable feelings during intercourse and orgasm takes time. A woman may find that the muscles at the entrance to her vagina are slacker. This reduces sensation during intercourse for both her and her partner. Doing the following exercises improves sensation – and makes for a better sex life.

Exercise

1. Squeeze the muscles around the vagina for three seconds, then relax for three seconds. Repeat 10 times. Do this three times a day.
2. Try to 'flutter' the vaginal muscles. Do 10 repeats, three times a day.

A woman can feel 'unsexy' for some time after childbirth. One woman spoke about avoiding sex because she felt so tired, haggard and lacking in passion. Sexual pleasure may seem like a long-lost memory when you feel dog-tired and crash into oblivion the moment your head hits the pillow at night. Your partner may be thrilled about becoming a father, but at the same time, threatened by the third person who, in his subconscious, may be a rival for your affections. He may want to have sex to re-establish your relationship and capture something special only you and he have. Don't be surprised if your partner is ready for sex before you are.

Feeling pressured into having sex, however, can make a woman resentful. Linden confided: *'I didn't feel like sex for ages. Even my husband's touch – which I usually enjoy – seemed distasteful. I was totally turned off.'*

CIRCLE THIS

Remember, even when you've recovered from the trauma of the birth and any stitches, you may experience some anxiety, and even fear, that sex will be painful. This may make you tense your vaginal muscles, making your fears a reality. It's best to share your feelings with your husband – and together build up desire and sexual activity between you slowly. By being sensitive to each other's needs, you'll both feel ready and sexy – but in your own time.

FEELING SEXY AGAIN

Working on feeling sexy again is important for your self-esteem and for your relationship. The following tips will help in your plan to regain sexual feelings:

Keep in touch

Remember, it's important to touch. Stay physically close. Just because you don't feel like sex, doesn't mean you can't touch one another. Keeping a physical connection – being affectionate with each other, is important. Giving and receiving welcomed touches affectionately, can help re-establish your physical relationship.

Kiss, cuddle and caress

Kissing, cuddling and caressing tells you you're loved and desired. It also tells your partner he is wanted and loved. Giving each other a sensual massage conveys strong messages. You don't have to have sex, but you can pleasure each other all over – tickling, teasing and caressing.

Keep time for you and your partner to relax and enjoy each other

Take time out from your busy routine to just relax and enjoy each other's company, without the distraction of children and other demands. You might think about flirting over a sumptuous, candle-lit dinner, or taking a long, fragranced bath together.

NOW FOR THE GOOD NEWS

Almost all women with birth blues get better with time. They can be greatly helped by friends, family members, an understanding doctor or counsellor or self-help group. However, it's hard to estimate the time needed for women to recover. It depends on how quickly a woman was diagnosed, how seriously she was post-natally depressed, how much support she received and the quality of the treatment she was given.

Some experts believe that usually women feel much better six months after their initial feelings of depression. But it's difficult to make generalisations. One recent study found that 50% of women who did not seek treatment, were still depressed six months later.

Fortunately, professional help has come a long way. Dr Marie-Paule Austin believes the correct approach to help post-natally depressed women is to understand the individual woman in her unique context. She says: *'In the past, treatment was a little too simplistic. We'd tend to focus on the mother only. Now we look at the whole picture. There's not much point curing the mother and leaving her unconnected with the baby. We check whether her relationship with her partner is good as well.'*

A woman is not alone. Usually there is a husband or partner in the picture. Recent studies have suggested that one of the single most important factors that offsets depressed feelings in women is the knowledge that they have support from their partner. So make sure you're getting what you need from your partner – it could spare you some of the birth blues – or at the very least, make you feel better about yourself and your role. After all, in today's world, it is unfair to expect you to go it alone. Remind him of how rewarding it can be to get involved in supporting you and helping around the home.

Post-natal depression is an acceptable, legitimate experience. Give yourself permission to ask for your partner's support. Join a women's group. Some local areas have follow-up groups for moms. Do something radical – start your own Meet-a-Mum group where mothers meet over coffee and chat about their concerns, anxieties and fears. Get a self-help group going – network, and share the child care. Develop a roster and start a Parent Support network. Make as many social contacts as you can – and if you're a stay-at-home mum – get out of the house as often as you can.

If your mom lives close-by, seek out her support and let her help you in practical ways. Let go of the embarrassment you might feel about looking to your mum for help – after all, she probably got some help in her day with you!

Clarissa, who spoke earlier about feeling jealous of her baby in the early days, found that the understanding and support she got from her husband, was the turning point for her,

'Having your first baby is not as easy as everyone makes out. It's got its side-effects and after-effects. It really affects your feelings. But I was fortunate to have an understanding husband who accepted my depression, didn't judge me and that gave me tremendous hope. It helped me believe in myself. I knew I could get better.'

Clarissa's point of 'believing in yourself' is a good one. Believing in yourself results in being kind to yourself. It helps you understand that things will get better.

CIRCLE THIS

Believe that things will get better. Look after the baby as best you can. Learn to look after yourself as well. Give yourself time. Try to do your own thing when you can. And accept help when it's offered. Don't be shy – ask for help when you need it and don't beat yourself up to get things done. Take Clarissa's advice here, *'Get a nappy service'* and Linden's *'Get plenty of sleep.'*

A final word: Offer support to other mothers you meet. Heed Marni's comment. Ask them what you would like asked of you, *'And how are you?'*

7
A BABY MAYBE

*You want a baby so much. You'd give up all sorts of things
to see your child grow to adulthood. You'd give up certain parts
of your body. Here, take an arm. Take a leg.*

HANNAH CHICOWSKI

For many women who are unable to conceive, post-natal depression may appear to be a small price to pay for a baby. Women who are childless often feel like they are missing out on an essential experience of womanhood. Hannah Chicowski's words convey the high emotions that wanting to be a mother carries.

When Carolyn speaks, I can hear the pain. She says:

'I feel so isolated from the rest of the world. Pregnancy is something other women work hard to avoid. I used to work at avoiding it before I found I had a fertility problem. Now, I feel different – here I am working hard, trying to conceive. It's a topsy-turvy world.

'I hear pregnant friends moaning about their fertility and the prospect of another child and I sit in clinic waiting rooms hoping that this time I'll be lucky and get pregnant. My self-esteem was very low and I got terribly depressed with all the technical procedures – and no results. But I joined a support group and I can now accept I am a whole woman – and I know I don't have to turn my anger and frustration on myself. But still, I can't help but feel a little blue about things at times – I guess it's only natural.'

Carolyn, a 39 year old teacher has come a long way over the four years she's invested in her quest for pregnancy. She has come to terms with the strong ambivalent feelings her condition inevitably stirs up and yet, part of her remains unreconciled to her fate.

She explains that she has given herself the benefit of one last chance on the GIFT programme. GIFT is the shortening for Gamete Intra-Fallopian Transfer, a procedure in which the woman's eggs are collected, but instead of being taken to the laboratory for fertilization (as in IVF or In-Vitro Fertilization), the eggs together with previously collected and washed sperm are placed directly into a normal fallopian tube using a fine sterile plastic tube.

Taking me back to the beginning of her story, Carolyn reveals a journey which has left her feeling depressed and searching for some explanation, knowing that it is unlikely she will ever find an adequate enough one. Carolyn has learned to live with fragments of understanding, moments of acceptance and times of continuing confusion and sadness.

Carolyn says that she fully expected to get pregnant, have children and live happily ever after. She had a life-plan mapped out and when she met her husband, Jack, 10 years ago, she knew he was the man with whom she intended making her plans a reality. After two years they decided to start a family. At first, they thought that in time Carolyn would get pregnant. They were in no rush and they had heard that it could take about a year after coming off the Pill for a woman to conceive.

But two years after Carolyn stopped taking the Pill, she still wasn't pregnant. This was the first time Carolyn entertained the idea – the fear – that something might be wrong. At the same time, she says she pushed this fear away, wanting to believe it wasn't really happening. After all, as Carolyn says, she believed she had a *'God-given right to have a baby'*. It was around this time that Carolyn says she began to feel depressed.

Another year and no pregnancy later, Carolyn and Jack were faced with the decision of seeking help. Carolyn admits it might have been easier to let things just drift along and hope for the best. But she felt she needed more information and more control. Though still feeling depressed, Carolyn says that she and Jack discussed their options and decided they wanted children. They decided to seek help.

The quest for a baby can be all-consuming. It's difficult for the childless couple to forget the latest dinner party – when everyone else was proudly showing pictures of their children – or the awkward silences that follow a seemingly innocent question like, 'Do you have children?'

For one in ten couples, the journey towards possible parenthood includes tests that turn their life around, or upside down. Even a calm woman can become a bundle of nerves as she hopes each month that her period will not come. It can strengthen a relationship or it has the potential to tear it apart. The impact of being infertile is a life crisis. It shakes your ideas about yourself, your femininity and it may involve a shift in your ideas about how your life will proceed. The journey to achieve a pregnancy is full of hope, promise and possible disappointment – and feelings of depression. If a woman seeks medical help, her life will suffer enormous intrusions. Personal life is open to scrutiny, tests and the inevitable strain on her relationship.

BACK TO THE BEGINNING

It all began with the birth of Louise Brown on 27 July 1978 at exactly 11.47 pm at Oldham District Hospital in England. Louise Brown's birth was a miracle bringing hope to many women living with infertility. Louise Brown was the first so-called 'test-tube baby'. She was the result of twelve years of intensive research by Drs Steptoe, a gynaecologist and Edwards, a physiologist.

Today, a dazzling array of fertility procedures and alternatives are available. IVF, GIFT, ZIFT, donor eggs, donor sperm, frozen embryos and surragacy offer women living with fertility options that were undreamed of twenty years ago. There are options for trying to conceive your own genetic child, to carrying a non-biological child to term, to having someone else carry a child for you through surrogacy. The reproductive technologies to assist conception all have one purpose – to help a woman have a baby.

From the woman's point of view, the available choices all offer her hope. Hope and possible triumph are what keeps the woman going. The success stories help to bolster hope in the face of unsuccessful attempts. The depth of wisdom that the experience of crisis which infertility brings also acts to sustain hope.

When Carolyn went on a fertility program she began to feel hopeful. But month after month, when no pregnancy resulted, she became more and more depressed. She also became obsessed with the idea of being 'incomplete'. She was missing something as a woman – a child. She said that everywhere she looked there were women with children and people asking her insensitive questions. She said,

> 'I'd be upset by questions like, 'How many children do you have?' And one day, I remember seeing a lot of pregnant women at the supermarket and bursting into tears, wondering if I'd ever be pregnant. It even got to the stage that I'd burst into tears at the sight of a pram or a pregnant woman. One Mother's Day, I burst into tears when a sales assistant asked me what my children had given me as presents.'

Other women echo Carolyn's words. They have experienced similar strong reactions when they see mothers and children or pregnant women. These women often say that they are confused – and ashamed of their reactions, yet they can't help their feelings – a mixture of envy, resentment, self-pity and despair.

Carolyn recognised she had an obsession, yet she was unable to do anything about it. In her words,

> 'I was gripped by a madness. I had to have my own genetic child. I would've done whatever it took. I had no moral problems with any of it. No cost – financial or emotional – was too great. I had to take some positive action. I told myself I had to stop avoiding the supermarket at certain hours because I couldn't face pregnant women with toddlers.'

PREGNANCY AS AN OBSESSIVE DESIRE

Like Carolyn, some women become obsessed with the idea of having a baby. Their attitude shifts from 'it'd be nice to have a baby' to 'if I don't have a baby, I'll die'. The intensity of emotions involved is overwhelming. The responsibility the woman feels for making the pregnancy happen is immense. Each time she 'fails' to conceive, she becomes anxious, frustrated, sad, angry and depressed. Many women report becoming totally obsessed with conception. They say they are taken over by it.

For Josephine, this obsessive desire and her chronic depression took over her life for three years. Each month for three years she was disappointed. Josephine, 37, is a copywriter and a woman who expected herself to cope with almost any adversity – she thought she was 'strong and capable'. In the face of infertility problems, she found she became 'weak, teary and depressed'. Josephine was accustomed to planning for and organising her life. Until she had trouble conceiving, she had managed to organise her life beautifully.

Missing a period is one of the first signs of pregnancy. Josephine's anxiety became focused on whether or not she'd miss her period. Josephine's period was a monthly reminder of her failure to get pregnant. After she went onto a fertility program, this monthly reminder was all the harder to accept. The regimen she followed was also depressing. She said:

> *I'd have a blood test at 7.00 am at the hospital and then go to work. In the afternoon, I'd go back for another injection. This injection was to help stimulate ovulation and the blood test showed how close to ovulating I was. This was my life over a period of 18 months for two-and-a-half weeks out of every month. You can imagine how draining it got. I almost gave up after the third month. I'd think I can't do this anymore. This is too hard. It was difficult trying to stay positive but not getting your hopes up too high. I knew I had to stay motivated. Deep down, I'd think, 'Yes, it's going to happen.' Then I'd think it wouldn't. Every time I got a period I'd die inside. But I had to keep thinking, 'Next time, next time.''*

This mantra of 'next time, next time' is at the heart of a poem written by Rhonda Relecker:

Maybe Next Time

Pregnant or not? – which was it to be?
The answer was "No" and my husband said to me
"Maybe next time."

I knew that he shared my grief, my loss
and I wondered if trying was worth the cost.
"Why not now? Why not us? I just can't cope."
But then I saw in his eyes the offer of hope.

Now I know that we both hope and pray
that it will happen, and we won't need to say
"Maybe next time."

Hope and obsession. And obsession leading to hope. And hope leading to obsession. Each woman wants to believe that her obsession will move beyond hope – and produce the sought-after reality: a baby.

A journalist, Annie Dodds, writes movingly about her obsession in the face of 'unexplained infertility'. She writes about all the advice given to her and her husband by well-meaning friends, the consultation with the psychic and the mail-order herbs:

> 'Emotionally fatigued from dealing with our infertility, Jeff and I decided to have a treatment-free year and travelled overseas for two months. Unfortunately, our emotional baggage travelled with us. By the time we arrived in Rome, I was in such a state of despair that I found myself praying for a baby on a pew in St Peter's. My momentary lapse in atheism amounted to nothing. Back home, we drifted unhappily until we were jolted into action by my birthday. I turned 35. Propelled by the feeling that we might have regrets later, we finally decided to try IVF. We were desperate and resigned to IVF being our only chance of ever having a baby. We knew it was a risky investment of hope, energy and money. The statistics on the success rate are grim – about 15 to 20 per cent... The nurse explained the procedures involved and concluded by saying: 'We take over your body.' If only she knew how frightening that sounded.'

In a society where motherhood is symbolically important and confirms women's female identity, childless women and those with reproductive problems are often asked to explain themselves. Women without children are seen as incomplete. Womanhood is seen as the ability to create, bear and nurture a child. When a woman has a child, she confirms for herself and others that she is a complete woman. Birth is celebrated. It is the only defence against the inevitability of death and offers new hope for the future.

Woman's special capacity to bear children is prized and celebrated. A woman unable to conceive misses out on this 'specialness'. Sylvia Plath wrote in her poem, *Childless Woman:*

The womb
Rattles its pod the moon
Discharges itself from the tree with nowhere to go.

Many women's plans for their future lives are often linked to expectations of becoming mothers. There is a common view that only women with children are 'proper' women, even in these times of public commitment to gender equality.

TABOOS AND SILENCE

Infertility is an extremely private problem. Often it is felt as shameful, something about which to be embarrassed. The search for a cure, the journey undertaken in the hope of achieving pregnancy is often embarrassing, involving grim, technical invasions into what should be a private and spontaneous encounter. As Annie Dodds was told, 'We take over your body'.

Yet, women who are infertile have to live in a fertile society. Marriage is a fertility rite. The happy young couple, despite modern talk about choice and contraception, are under constraint to reproduce. Expressions such as 'Orange blossom this year, orange juice next' and 'May all your troubles be little ones', suggest that the young couple have no way out. If they don't reproduce quickly, people around them feel entitled to ask questions.

It is true to say that the majority of couples get married with every expectation of having children. Some women, therefore, experience a state of childlessness, of not being a mother, as a personal failure.

In ***Who's Afraid of Virginia Woolf?***, Edward Albee explores this theme of childlessness. George and Martha are on trial for the childlessness of their marriage and its implications for family life. In the play, George and Martha play an ageing college professor and his wife who play host to a new, young college professor, Nick and his wife, Honey. Nick confides in George that Honey has had a hysterical or imaginary pregnancy. He says, *'She blew up and then she went down.'* George casually asserts, *'Martha doesn't have pregnancies at all.'*

George and Martha's relationship is a love/hate one which has witty repartee and much verbal violence. Although they throw hostility and hatred at one another, they also turn immediately to each other for emotional support.

Albee deftly demonstrates the folie à deux that George and Martha are caught up in. The two of them have maintained the illusion of a son to compensate for Martha's never having any children to give their seemingly empty lives some content. With the death of their imaginary son, comes the death of their neurotic way of life. It symbolises a ritualistic rebirth of themselves.

Who's Afraid of Virginia Woolf?, a play written in 1962 and made famous on the screen with performances by Elizabeth Taylor and Richard Burton, contains messages ahead of its time. Yet, even today, the same issues Albee addresses are relevant.

Feminists have written about their surprise to find that taboos and silence around infertility are as strong in the women's movement as elsewhere. These taboos and silence have made many women angry, sad and depressed. The woman with fertility problems, her experiences and needs remain largely invisible.

What is also invisible is the grief. Not being able to conceive is rather like having a child die. In some ways a woman may experience it as worse because it seems difficult to mourn the loss of something that didn't happen. But understanding the grief and giving voice to the experience is necessary if women are to feel empowered.

Women seeking motherhood, pursuing motherhood with all their might must be allowed a voice. Joy, 42, has been on the emotional roller-coaster for many years. Her voice is heard in the following comment,

> 'I seem to be surrounded by women who have children. They have a choice, whereas I have no choice. I feel so vulnerable to strong emotions. I hate feeling so envious, so judgemental but you have to understand how angry and sad I feel. I believe all women should have the right to choose to have an abortion, for instance. But, it breaks my heart, when I'm so desperate to become pregnant – to hear about women who don't want their pregnancy, or are having abortions or tubal ligations. Sometimes I feel alone – like I'm the only one who doesn't have the luxury of choice.'

This voice can often be hopeful and positive and sometimes it can be sad, low, negative and depressed. It is this negative voice which is hard to listen to – but nevertheless, needs to be heard. Women should have our permission to tell us how hard it is for them.

Women, and men alike, should also have our permission to tell us how hard it is for them as a couple to survive the crisis of infertility.

WHAT'S HAPPENING TO OUR RELATIONSHIP?

It is often difficult for the couple to cope with the powerful emotions that infertility raises in their relationship. Anger, guilt and depression can grow in intensity unless the couple are vigilant about keeping the effects of these emotions at bay.

Relationships can be seen as a system – with interaction continually occurring between partners. What affects one person will, in time, affect their spouse. For instance, the stresses on one spouse and the behaviour that results affects the actions of their partner and ultimately, the condition of their relationship. Mostly, it is the woman who must face the invasive testing and treatments. She might begin to feel that her husband is not sharing the burden.

He, in turn might be feeling vulnerable and unable to share his feelings.

Throwing himself into work and withdrawing from the relationship results in both parties feeling like they don't understand each other. Alternatively, the man might be resentful and angry that he has to 'perform' sexually and on demand. Some men have spoken angrily about feeling like 'sexual robots'. In turn, the woman might begin to feel that her husband is not as concerned in trying to conceive. She might feel hurt and unable to discuss her fears. Again, the end result is that both parties retreat – and become self-protective. They find they struggle to communicate in a rational and reasonable manner. What began for them as a committed and focused journey towards parenthood has the potential to end up with the couple struggling to salvage the broken fragments of their relationship.

CIRCLE THIS

Remember, it's normal for infertility to cause stress in your relationship. It's how you deal with it that counts.

HOW DOES A COUPLE SURVIVE THIS TESTING TIME?

Tips for survival

- Make an effort to communicate–your affection, your humour, your sexuality
- Maintain a sense of appreciation for the good points in your partner and the strengths in your relationship
- Don't be an 'ostrich' about problems as they arise – face them and deal with them before they overwhelm you and your relationship
- Share your thoughts and emotions with each other – no matter how fearful you might be
- Accept the fact that you and your partner are individuals – and as different people, you will inevitably respond differently to things that happen
- Be willing to rekindle your feelings for one another and renew your closeness, by planning a vacation from treatment – and preferably away from your home and your routine
- Agree together on a time limit for undergoing infertility treatment – and then try to keep to it

Most importantly, consider going for counselling as a couple. Counselling can help you address the emotions raised by infertility and help you work through any blocks which may be affecting your relationship. Counselling can also help open up the block the couple may have in talking openly about their infertility. It is often in counselling also, that the couple come to realise that their survival as a couple may mean deciding on an end point to infertility programs. This end point may well restore balance and sanity to their lives – and act to strengthen their relationship.

THE END OF THE BABY CHASE

There comes a time for all couples when they have to accept their childlessness. This is a particularly difficult time for a woman. Extinguishing all hope is hard.

However, a woman can help herself by understanding that she has to grieve. She grieves all the babies she's never had. She needs to have understanding people who will listen to her and help her to resolve her pain.

Fenella's 10 year obsession to have children ended with her hysterectomy. She became severely depressed after her operation and went into therapy for two years. She said:

> 'I had my hopes dashed every month when I got my period. Then I went on IVF but I wasn't one of the lucky ones. I couldn't believe Mother Nature could be so cruel – I was stunned when the doctor told me I would lose my womb. I got so depressed I thought I would rather die than face life without children and no hope of ever having any.'

Fenella said she found it helpful when people could say, 'I think I understand'. Finding understanding and supportive people is crucial if the woman is to grieve and find resolution.

Through therapy, Fenella learned that her baby chase was over, but the rest of her life was just beginning. Fenella had put so much effort into her baby chase, yet it hadn't paid off. Her need to accept life without her own genetic child was important in order for her to move on with her life.

Another woman, Nicola, found giving up the quest to have her own child painful. But she knew it was part of her journey. She said:

> 'We put everything into it. I put my life on hold for two years, but it wasn't meant to be. We were prepared to try everything and anything. I have to say that it was like I was obsessed for a while, but like everything, you can't keep going forever. There's so much grief involved – I was pregnant twice, but then I lost them both – I couldn't keep going. After my last attempt, which wasn't successful, I knew I couldn't try again. It started interfering with my life, our relationship – we'd become one-tracked – constant talk about doctors, drugs, operations, hopes, depression and constant fear of failure. I decided enough was enough. We'd tried our best. I'd given up some of my life for this. It was time to continue the rest of my life.'

Culturally, it's difficult for a woman to say 'no' to further technology. And Nicola attests to this. She had many attempts on a fertility program and finally decided she could not proceed. The increase in options in reproductive technology makes the pressure not to say 'no' even greater than before. Under what circumstances can a woman say no?

Vanessa, 41, describes herself as a 'veteran' of reproductive technology. She finally said 'no' because the seductiveness of trying something new with a 'better' success rate was starting to interfere with what she called her 'integrity as a person'. She could not live with a constant dangling of carrots, the enticement to try something new, if the technology did not work. She felt she couldn't keep trying one program after another and remain 'human'. She wanted her 'body and life back' and believed the cost of becoming a 'reproductive technology junkie' was too great a price to pay.

The 'getting on with one's life' theme runs through narratives given by women who have decided to say 'no' to further attempts. One woman revealed: *'I couldn't face failure anymore. It was taking too much emotional energy. The pain of being on the program was greater than the pain of being childless'.*

ARE YOU READY TO STOP TRYING?

When to stop trying? Try answering the following questions honestly:

- Do you hate the idea of fertility programs taking over your life?
- Does the prospect of no more thermometers, drugs and doctors' appointments sound like heaven?
- Have you exhausted all known medical possibilities?
- Do you dislike the kind of person you've become – obsessed, tired, irritable and depressed?
- Do you dream of recapturing happiness as a 'normal couple'?
- Is the pain of being on the program greater than the pain of being childless?
- Are you ready to consider adoption?
- Are you prepared for a childfree life?

Look at your responses. If you answered 'yes' to a majority of the questions, then it's probably safe to say that you are ready to stop trying.

Many women have found formalising their decision to not proceed with the baby chase brought with it a sense of resolution. Letting go and saying goodbye to your genetic child is important. From the feeling of depression can come feelings of being at peace and a sense of calm.

By replacing unfulfilled dreams with reality, the woman can begin to feel comfortable with her future. It is at this point that the woman – and indeed, the couple – are ready to get on with their lives – to decide to adopt, or to live childfree.

THE POWER OF RITUAL

By performing a ritual around the decision to say 'no' to further attempts, a woman can put closure on her baby chase. One woman who benefitted from performing a ritual to mark the end of her attempts to conceive is Vanessa, who spoke earlier. Vanessa said,

> *'I can still remember the counsellor telling me I should do something to mark the end of my attempt to have my own baby. She suggested I include my husband in this. So my husband and I talked about it and we came up with the idea of writing down our hopes and our disappointments and putting it in*

> *a bottle which could float out to sea. It was a very cleansing thing to do – I can still see that bottle bobbing around and moving away from us – and finally it was invisible. That marked the end for us – and it was a great release.'*

This sense of a 'great release' is shared by other women who have formalized and ritualized the end of their baby chase. They have all done it in their own unique and different way. They all designed a meaningful event.

Rituals are events which help provide meaning and give structure to our lives. They can be cleansing and releasing. They usually involve catharsis. Catharsis provides a relief of the emotions. It performs a cleansing or ridding function – and one which leaves a person feeling better about themselves and their lives. And ready to move on.

The ritual around giving up hoping means letting go of the seductive whisper of 'miracles can happen' – and the moving on to an acceptance of an end to hope. Rituals can also serve to release the bottled-up grief. Rituals can heal – and prevent that delayed shock that some women report feeling, after believing they had come to terms with their childlessness.

Rituals heal and provide an outlet for the couple – as partners in grief. Another woman, Agnes, shared her ritual, which involved creativity and imagination. Agnes suggested to her husband that they paint a wooden box together in the colours and images that represented their journey and destination. She comments,

> *'At first Jim was a little apprehensive, but we started working on the box slowly. We began by using neutral, safe colours and then we got bolder and more dramatic. That box was our art, our work-in-progress, it symbolized our thoughts, feelings and actions. We'd always work on it together, this was a joint enterprise. When we finished, the box looked beautiful, it was colourful and we'd painted images important to us – rainbows, trees, cats, fruit and of course, babies. We were so moved by the finished product – it was our work – it was our baby.'*

Agnes goes on to say that she and Jim couldn't leave the inside of the box plain. So they lined it with rich blue velvet. Then they decided to keep the box in their living room. They wanted to be able to see and touch the box, which had taken on magical qualities of reassurance and new hope for the future for them.

It is important for the woman – and the couple – to perform their own ritual when they are ready. They must do something that makes sense for them. Remember, this ritual is very individualistic. Maybe it's the message in the bottle like it was for Vanessa, or maybe it's the making of a box symbolising your hopes and struggles and sense of acceptance, or maybe it's something totally different.

Lawrence Baron, a professor of history at San Diego State University, and his wife Bonnie, a clincial social worker told Sherry Suib Cohen in *New Woman*, that they wanted to mark and mourn the death of their dream of having a biological child. They decided they needed a ceremony to share their feelings with others. A support group of 55 people – relatives and friends, were invited to share and bear witness to the Barons' acceptance of their childlessness. They wrote a service which was filled with poetry and music. It was a healing service sharing their deepest feelings. Bonnie said,

> '*We wrote down our regrets and our hopes. When the day came, we went down to the ocean, surrounded by our friends and family, and we threw symbols of our regrets into the sea.*'
>
> '*There is an ancient Jewish ceremony for mourners in which a black ribbon worn on the mourner's clothing is cut, a symbol of anger and grief: because we could not know the gender of our unborn children, we wore little pink and blue ribbons, mourning the loss of unborn lives.*'

Lawrence claimed that from that day, they stopped trying to have a baby. He said,

> '*It felt wonderful. We buried the idea, grieved for it, and finished with it. Now, we can decide whether to adopt or stay childless. We can move ahead.*'

CIRCLE THIS

Whatever you decide on as a ritual, you'll have a marker that's going to help you heal the wounds of having one important choice in life taken from you.

THE ADOPTION OPTION

Adoption as an option is viable for the woman who has resolved her depression and decided to not remain childfree. For some women, and men, it's imperative to become a parent. That role of parent is so important for some women, that they must have it, no matter what. Adopting, is an individual matter which needs to be researched thoroughly.

Understanding your motivations

To adopt means taking on the responsibility of parenting another person's biological child. If a woman wants to become a mother at all costs, then her motivation to adopt is clear. However, the first step is evaluation by the woman, and this is essential. If she discovers that the experience of pregnancy and birth are important, then the adoption option is questionable. Likewise, if a woman, in her evaluation, discovers that she really had a burning desire to carry on family traits, then adoption will fail to meet her needs.

Before turning to the option of adoption, each woman should carefully examine her life, her needs and wants, and only when she is clear on all these – should she make the decision to apply for adoption.

CIRCLE THIS

There is such a phenomenon as 'postadoption blues'. The experience of adopting can be overwhelming, and abrupt. Although the adopted child is much wanted, many women overlook the possibility of some low feelings – anxiety, irritability and depression. Of course, these are normal responses to a sudden change in your life, but the reality is, these changes are emotionally demanding.

We live in a culture in which couples are expected to have children. It can be difficult – and in some cases, impossible – to go against the norm.

Fortunately, the Brave New World of reproductive technologies offers an ever increasing and confronting array of options. Surrogacy and donor-egg programs mean that every woman can have a child – if that is her wish. These non-genetic children can still fulfill a woman's dreams of becoming a mother. Nevertheless, there will be a certain proportion of women who will decide to remain childfree.

LIVING CHILDFREE – 'IT'S NOT THE END OF THE WORLD'

There are many advantages to living childfree, and truly accepting childlessness. The woman can console herself that she can find new satisfactions in her life. She will feel she has been strengthened by her experience and come full circle – from hope about becoming a mother to new hope for herself as a person.

CIRCLE THIS

What a woman has gained in her experience of infertility cannot be easily undone. Just as she experienced happy times in the past, so there will be happy times in the future. In fact, her experiences act to strengthen her perspective on life – and help her fashion a new happiness celebrating all her attempts and the new chapter in her life.

It is important to look at the happy events in your life and not focus on not having children. Reframing can help here.

A NOTE ON REFRAMING

Have you ever noticed how two women who observe the same event, such as a baseball game will give different descriptions of what happened? Each woman's picture, painted from her own perspective, will have a frame that is appropriate for that woman with her own particular viewpoint.

The idea behind reframing is not to deny the way you see the world, but to offer an expanded view of the world.

Reframing provides the woman with an expanded picture of her world. This expanded picture enables her to perceive her situation differently – and more constructively.

So, instead of feeling down because you can't take your daughter to her ballet class – think how lucky you are to have the time to pursue your own tap class!

You don't have to be a total Pollyanna – but it really does help to reflect on the positive.

Take note: Look at the list below. Rejoice in your childfree life-style and think how good it feels that:

- you can enjoy the spontaneity and joie de vivre that having a normal sex life offers – free of thermometers, injections and implanting
- you'll never have to think, 'this is the night' – which has started having you feel that sex is something you have to do to get the baby you desperately want
- no more sex-on-schedule for 'maximum fertility opportunity' – and no more waning passion and sex regimented by the calendar
- the monthly disappointment no longer need overshadow the good things in life
- infertility teaches a woman she can get through a serious crisis

Remember that as a woman – and a couple – you have survived a process that is traumatic – and that is worthy of commendation in and of itself.

Many couples find that their relationship is strengthened and they feel wiser for their journey. They may feel closer to each other, because they've learned about themselves and each other. They have survived individually. And they have survived as a couple. That is commendation indeed.

'LIFE IS TERRIFIC NOW'

Women can enjoy a fertile life without children. The words of Robert Frost, resonate for those women whose lives have taken a less usual path:

The Road Not Taken

'Two roads diverged in a wood, and I –
I took the one less traveled by,
And that has made all the difference'

The metaphor of a journey, away from a sense of loss, towards something more positive emerged in discussions with childless women. What appears to happen is that after women confront and start to work through childlessness, they begin to feel they can own their own life. The woman is free to take on board her own unique variety of living – not necessarily the one she is expected to assume. She begins to understand her place in the world. She knows she must fashion out her own life. She has her own truth.

Childfree living can hold as much day-to-day purpose as living with children. A productive life is possible. In Josephine's words *'Life is terrific now'*. She and her husband are living childfree and enjoying it. Life without children has meant more time, freedom and money. Josephine has one piece of advice to women contemplating life without children, *'Ignore the women's magazines and their message of children as necessary for a full life'*. Vanessa has another message, *'Regain control and be clear about what you want to do with your life. Make the most of all your talents and opportunities.'*

The final word goes to Agnes:

> *'My life is rich in many ways. I have an interesting job and I've traveled extensively. My husband and I have outside interests and an active social life. I'm very close to my two sisters and their daughters. I've become a positive role model for my three nieces.'*

POSTSCRIPT

Eighteen months after my interview with Carolyn, I received a letter. Carolyn's obsession had paid off. Her story of her five year struggle had come to an end. Carolyn writes:

> *'I would like to share my story of ultimate success with you. Over the five years on the program I never really felt like giving up, but I did get very depressed. On my twelfth go – I fell pregnant, and two months ago, I had a dear little girl. After those torrid years, my pregnancy was easy and the birth normal. I don't know why I was one of the lucky ones but here are my tips – things that I believe helped me in the last couple of cycles:*
>
> - *very little alcohol and no smoking*
> - *a good daily multivitamin, folic acid tablet and a blood cleanser such as Dong Quai or Chlorella*
> - *plenty of rest*
> - *keeping my sense of humour*

- *not dwelling on disappointments*
- *getting on with life and trying to stay busy*
- *meeting other women on the program to exchange ideas, theories, shed some tears and have a laugh*
- *supportive parents and friends*
- *a loving husband*

I can't tell you how ecstatic I was when my doctor said those hoped-for words to me, 'Congratulations, you're pregnant'. I'll cherish those words forever. I wish everyone on a fertility program the best of luck. And share my news with women you meet – waiting for their turn to come around. It does happen. It happened to me.'

8

WHEN A MOTHER LOSES A CHILD

*I have come to the conclusion, after many years
of sometimes sad experience, that you cannot come to any
conclusion at all.*

VITA SACKVILLE-WEST

Certainly for any mother, or for that matter, any parent who loses a child, it is hard to come to a sensible conclusion. No under-standable conclusion exists. Losing a child is devastating. It is unfathomable. So many emotions crowd into a woman's mind.

But, it is the intense sense of loss which is at the root of the emotions and confusion.

A woman can feel nothing – or she might feel like an emotional volcano. Anger, rage, bitterness, shame, guilt, despair and depression might all be experienced – in a single day or a single hour.

Gloria Vanderbilt, in writing about the impact the death of her son Carter had on her said: *'The losses in my life over the years had been many, each loss stripping me down to another layer, bringing me closer to the centre of myself. But the loss of Carter had not stripped off another layer – it had exploded the core of what I had known myself to be, and a new self would have to be born if I were to survive.'* Gloria Vanderbilt did two things: she critically analysed the circumstances of Carter's death, in order to bring some measure of understanding to the trauma. She also started writing letters to Carter. In these letters, she tried to make sense of the tragedy of Carter's death and revealed her excruciating pain. Gloria Vanderbilt echoed Vita Sackville-West's sentiments, when she wrote: *'I don't understand anything anymore. All I understand is pain.'*

Many women, like Gloria Vanderbilt, try to make sense of the loss of their child. They search for a cause, a meaning that will make the pain easier to bear. It's difficult to understand the death of your child because it goes against the natural order of things. By having a child die, a mother is confronted by an seemingly illogical reality. She needs to readjust to this ultimate shock. Moira, a 56 year old was shocked by the accidental death of her 27 year old daughter. She said,

> *'It didn't seem possible – she had the right to survive me – she was my daughter. She was this unique individual and I loved her very much. Suddenly she was taken from me. For a long time I was in a daze, a sort of denial about her death. I was very depressed and my grieving happened over about two years. Sometimes I thought it would never end. I still miss her terribly.'*

Searching for causes and seeking to identify why your child died is a common response. Women are particularly vulnerable following the unexplained death of a baby. Some women become obsessive about their need to understand the reason for what happened. Patrice, 28 was one such woman. She experienced a stillbirth. It had been her first pregnancy, which she had planned. She said,

> *'It was all so vague. I was left wondering what had happened. Why had what happened happen? The doctor wasn't sure why. I was just mad with wanting to know why. I started to wonder about the justice of it all. I mean, drug addicts have healthy babies. And alcoholic women have healthy babies. I remember being so careful, I took care of myself. I didn't drink coffee and I exercised in moderation. I did everything I could to make for a good pregnancy, but how much control do we have anyway? It really challenged my beliefs about doing the right thing.'*

Many women have talked about their beliefs being shaken and their trust in the world lost until they came to their own unique understanding and acceptance of the loss of their child.

At the turn of the last century, it was common for a woman to lose several children. The saying, 'In the midst of life we are in death' was an all-too-literal one. Today, we are not as familiar with the uncompromising face of childhood death. Environmental conditions and medical advances have meant better living conditions and longer life.

Today, we expect to lead relatively healthy and long lives. The death of our children is traumatic because we don't expect them to die before us. For instance, infant mortality has been cut so drastically that people are less prepared to cope with it than 50 years ago. Some women have spoken about their sense of personal failure (whether or not the failure is warranted) and their belief that most people have very little idea of what it is like to lose a child.

Surviving the loss of your child is a major life event. For those women who are confronted by this loss, Gloria Vanderbilt's words may resound clearly: *'I don't understand anything anymore. All I understand is pain.'*

The loss a mother feels when her child dies is profound. No experience she has had can adequately prepare her for the emotions she feels after the loss of her child. Many claim that the loss of a child, and particularly of a baby, is felt far more intensely by the mother. This loss signifies the breaking of a powerful bond. The bond between mother and child develops very early. Often it is thought that this bond begins at birth. However, research findings tell us that this bond develops and deepens throughout a woman's pregnancy. Some women have said that their relationship with their child began before the birth. For some women, this relationship begins before the conception. In studies women have talked about how they have a 'representation' or idea in their minds about how a future baby might look, what their personality will be and how they will be as mother to the child. Some women fantasize or dream about pregnancy and becoming pregnant – and even the baby well before any decision is taken to have a child.

Women imagine what their child will be like and they have hopes and dreams for their unborn child. In this way, a woman subtly begins to form an attachment to her future child. Often women are not aware of how important – and how much a part of their lives – the future child has become. But, if you've ever listened to pregnant women in conversation you'll hear them speculating about the sex of the baby, names they have chosen, and rechosen, ideas about who the baby will look like and hopes for the baby's future. Maybe you'll recall being pregnant and being preoccupied with these thoughts – and sharing them with other women.

BONDING AND ATTACHMENT

We now know that human beings are born with the capacity to relate. Bonding and attachment are powerful elements which are at the centre of the mother-child connection. Bonding is the process of attachment between a child and mother. Not only representations of the baby, but an early form of bonding with the baby can begin even before conception. Attachment develops as a consequence of a mother's responsiveness to her baby's inherent tendency to seek closeness and be in a relationship with her. In fact, by the end of their first year, most children have developed a strong attachment, usually to one or both of their parents. If the baby is separated from the parent for even a short time, they become temporarily distressed.

Researchers have observed that even at ten weeks of age, a baby will not only prefer her mother's face, but will also be sensitive to any expression of emotion by the mother. Babies have been observed to show interest and happiness when their mothers smile, and to appear upset, angry and startled when she is angry. Interestingly, although at six months, the faces of strangers were experienced as neutral, by nine months, they are seen as negative. This means that substitutions in care-giving are more difficult to negotiate. It appears that around seven to nine months, what is called 'focused attachment' becomes evident. The baby becomes increasingly able to recognise her mother or attachment figure and to make sense of her – her actions, feelings and intentions can be read and anticipated.

According to John Bowlby, the famous theorist and researcher, elements of parenting and mothering are pre-programmed. Strong feelings are aroused in mothers in matters which concern their children. What has been called 'maternal sensitivity' has been described as the mother's ability and willingness to see and interpret her baby's behaviour and emotional states from the baby's point of view and respond appropriately. Mostly, mothers will soon recognise and react to their baby's signals. The mother's voice might be softer, her pitch higher as she soothes a crying baby. As any mother knows, paying attention to, talking and cuddling all help to soothe a baby's distress.

As the mother and child interact, their behaviour helps build a strong relationship between them. This relationship is very much a two-way phenomenon.

When a child dies, this bonding and the years of attachment behaviour are abruptly severed. Coming to terms with the death of your child is very traumatic. Your relationship with your child has been built up over the years and it has come to represent many things for you. Likewise, losing a child will also represent many things for you.

WHAT LOSING A CHILD REPRESENTS

Researchers have found that apart from the loss of the unique individual who was your child, you are likely to be affected by the absence of what your child represented to you. For instance, your child may have represented several, or maybe all of the following things:

- part of yourself – you remember your child's conception, and any characteristics that resemble you and your partner
- your source of love – your love was based on need, interdependence and appreciation
- your missed expectations – experiences you anticipated sharing with your child will never happen. The younger the child, the more anticipation and expectations you had about him or her.
- a loss of your power – you feel powerless and frustrated at not being able to exert more control over your child's fate.
- your connection with the future – your sense of continuity in the world was embodied in your child. The two of you were moving forward together in the coming years.

Jocelyn, 44, whose son died of a drug overdose at 16, spoke of her loss and what it represented in the following comment,

> 'My son was so much a part of my future, and now that he's gone, I'm not the same person. I loved him with my heart – and I know he loved me. He wanted so much from life, but he seemed to be in too much of a hurry. I wish I'd known how many risks he was taking. Maybe I could have convinced him to slow down. As it is, we've both lost the future.'

Children are the next generation. They are the link to the future. Maybe you've heard the old saying, 'Lose your parent and you've lost the past; lose your spouse and you've lost the present; lose your child and you've lost your future'. And maybe you believe there's a lot of truth in it.

CIRCLE THIS

For a mother, the loss of a child is the loss of a child, no matter what the child's age.

Dr Ronald Knapp who researched how parents coped with the death of a child, found that apart from some normal variability, parents have six frequent reactions to their loss.

First, parents, especially mothers, have a strong desire to never forget their child. Mothers are frightened that their memories of their child will fade with time.

Secondly, many parents needed to talk about their loss, and to share their feelings. However, this may not happen. Sometimes people feel too vulnerable to share their feelings, and sometimes they don't want to 'upset' others by talking about highly emotional matters. As Dr Knapp concluded, however, it is important for parents who are grieving to share their feelings and to seek out open and constructive communication with people they feel they can trust.

Thirdly, parents are often left thinking, 'Why not me? Why my child?' Feelings of absolute desolation and difficulty in accepting their own continuing life are strong, particularly in the first two weeks to three months after loss. Often, parents adopt a nonchalant attitude to death. In fact, Dr Knapp found that many parents who have children die, develop a permanent characteristic: they have no fear of death. Mothers, in particular, can become apathetic towards life – and often withdraw from life: they become depressed.

Fourthly, a majority of parents try to find some plausible reason for their loss. The mother tries to make sense of her experience, like Gloria Vanderbilt. Some parents turn to religion for answers and comfort. For some mothers, the experience of loss can result in a personal religious revival or conversion.

Fifthly, Dr Knapp believes that parents who have lost their children experience a shift in values. Traditional values and goals of our society might be questioned – why strive for personal success, when there are more intangible values that are more important? Some mothers refocused their sense of priority – family goals became more important than individual and career goals. Some women have spoken of a decreased concern with appearances and material possessions. For many parents, a loss leads to a heightened sense of vulnerability – and this leads to viewing life and time as more precious. Experiencing the loss of a child often has the consequence of making the mother more tolerant of others. She becomes more sensitive to and empathic with others and their problems.

Finally, many families who have lost are left with 'shadow grief'. This is the sort of grief that doesn't dominate, but even in time, is never completely forgotten. This grief can be prompted even by small reminders – and it produces anxiety, sadness and crying.

CIRCLE THIS

Moving from these confused and confusing feelings – and a sense of depression – through to resolution is the grieving journey. Achieving resolution is very much an individual matter. No-one can tell you how long it should take – nor should anyone sit in judgement on you. Don't expect yourself to be back 'to normal' in any particular length of time. And don't take on messages from people around you such as 'no use dwelling on the past' and 'well, life has to go on' and 'no use feeling sorry for yourself, you've got to start again'. Grieving takes place in a unique manner. You are the expert in your own grief. It takes as long as it needs to for you to feel better and move on – all in your own good time.

Take note: The death of a child can place enormous strain on the parents' relationship. The divorce rate following such bereavement is twice the national average for marital breakdown. Often parents are so shocked and stressed that they retreat into themselves. They may even unconsciously withdraw their love from their other children, fearful of reliving the agony should one of them die.

Siblings of the deceased child may also react by withdrawing. They are traumatised by the experience, and sometimes, by their parents' reaction. They may become clingy and anxious. Or they may react by becoming resentful. This resentment is sometimes expressed in outbursts of bad behaviour. Sometimes they may even feel responsible for – and guilty about their sibling's death.

Family members may be so preoccupied with their own grief that they are unable to deal with each other's sense of loss and depression. What sometimes ends up happening is that each family member is alone with her or his grief.

Mothers often believe it's their duty to provide all the support and nurturing in times of crisis. Yet, this expectation is unrealistic in the face of their own feelings of loss. Seeking help outside the family circle can help to exorcise the silent resentment corroding family relationships.

By finding support outside the family, you can come back to the family feeling refreshed and restored. This support can be obtained from friends – or better still, through professional counsellors and therapists. The sense of isolation that grief bestows on us can also be overcome with peer support from self-help groups.

The sense of loss a mother feels may be different, but no less intense, when she experiences the loss of a baby. Miscarriages, stillbirths and neonatal deaths raise some common issues for a mother. All of these deaths involve babies who have not yet been recognised by others. They have not been given a 'place' in society.

Unfortunately, many people make the mistake of believing that unless the child had a personality and a presence that was observed by others, the mother's grief is not as great as it would be had she lost an older child.

Often this lack of acknowledgement and sympathy from others deprives a mother of the understanding, affection and much-needed support.

AN UNACKNOWLEDGED LOSS

A startling 15% to 25% of early pregnancies end in loss. A miscarriage is an event that many women will face at some point in their reproductive life. Yet, as with infertility, perhaps even more so, there is still a conspiracy of silence around this event. Technically, a miscarriage means 'the expulsion of a foetus from the womb before 28 weeks of pregnancy'.

Too many people still regard miscarriage as a non-event. There are no traditional rituals or rites to mark the event. Well-intentioned comments can sometimes be heard as trivializing remarks, 'Don't worry, you'll soon have others'.

Miscarriage is usually followed by a deep emotional reaction. Many women are quite unprepared for the intensity of their feelings. Because bonding begins pre-birth, women who have their pregnancy abruptly ended, often with little warning, are left feeling acute anxiety and sorrow.

Women have reported their intense feelings – their guilt and self-reproach following a miscarriage. They blame themselves for miscarrying. They might ask, *'Am I ready to become a mother?'* They tell themselves they must be defective because they couldn't carry the baby to term. They blame the miscarriage on the fact that they kept on smoking, or drinking, or exercising or working too hard or having sex with their partners.

Their guilt is heard in the questions they ask their doctors: *'Why did it happen?' 'Was it something I did that I shouldn't have done?'* or *'Was is something that I didn't do that I should have done?'*

Unfortunately, women may never receive an answer that makes sense. There is no understandable conclusion. About 60% of miscarriages are caused by chromosomal abnormalities in the foetus, while the remaining 40% are unknown. If the doctor is unable to provide a specific reason for the miscarriage, it only adds to the woman's anxiety, confusion and feelings of depression.

Sylvia Plath wrote about these intense and confusing emotions in *Three Women: a Poem for Three Voices*:

I am not ugly. I am even beautiful.
The mirror gives back a woman without deformity.
The nurses give back my clothes, and an identity.
It is usual, they say, for such a thing to happen.
It is usual in my life, and the lives of others.
I am one in five, something like that. I am not hopeless.
I am beautiful as a statistic. Here is my lipstick.

I draw on the old mouth.
The red mouth I put by with my identity
A day ago, two days, three days ago. It was a Friday.
I do not even need a holiday; I can go to work today.
I can love my husband, who will understand.
Who will love me through the blur of my deformity,
As if I had lost an eye, a leg, a tongue.

And so I stand, a little sightless. So I walk
Away on wheels, instead of legs, they serve me well.
And learn to speak with fingers, not a tongue.
The body is resourceful.
The body is a starfish can grow back its arms.
And newts are prodigal in legs. And may I be
As prodigal in what lacks me.

Depression may be an inevitable part of the mourning and healing process for many women who experience a miscarriage.

Carissa, a 32 year old woman was shocked by the blasé attitude she encountered after her miscarriage at 14 weeks,

'Until I miscarried, I had no idea how common it is. I feel the whole topic needs to be publicised more – and people, especially women, need to be better educated. I was shocked by the medical and nursing staff treating the whole thing so lightly. They didn't seem to be aware of the emotional

after-effects. They said things like, 'you're young enough to try again' and 'you'll soon get over it' in such a breezy way. I didn't feel there was any recognition of the lost baby. It was as if the baby had never been conceived and therefore it didn't matter.'

As a result of her experience, Carissa said she became determined to read everything she could get her hands on, to inform herself. She said she received another shock to find there wasn't much available that would help her understand her experience intellectually, nor to help her heal emotionally.

Likewise, Lydia, 27, did not feel consoled by people she expected to understand. She miscarried at 26 weeks. She was told 'it was all for the best',

'I found it frustrating that the medical reasons for why I miscarried weren't clear. The doctors said different things, so it was confusing. I didn't know what to think and I got very depressed. I also had a lot of guilt because when I found out I was pregnant my husband was upset and accused me of duping him into starting a family before he was ready. I thought maybe I'd done something to jeopordize my baby – you know, unconsciously. Anyway, by the time I miscarried my husband had quite adjusted to the idea and he was really upset. I guess it's just that a woman can get so emotional at a time like that. All sorts of strange ideas get into your head. But it did hurt when one doctor said, 'A miscarriage is nature's way of sparing you an imperfect baby' – I can tell you that comment was very cold comfort.'

Women's reactions to miscarriage vary. They vary according to the time in pregnancy when the miscarriage occurs. They vary according to previous experience such as problems in pregnancy. And they vary according to the emotional investment the woman has in the particular pregnancy.

For instance, if a woman has a long history of infertility and she becomes pregnant and miscarries, she may well feel down about the experience, yet at another level more philosophical. One woman to whom this happened said, *'Well, I thought to myself, you can do it! I was worried because I was so sick during the pregnancy and I was scared the baby would be abnormal. And finally I thought, if I could do it once, I could get pregnant again.'* By contrast, another woman, already the mother of two children confided,

'The miscarriage was a terrible experience. I wondered 'why me?' I had this feeling of shame at not being able to produce a baby. After all, I'd had two.' For this woman, the idea of miscarriage had never crossed her mind. One wonders whether it had crossed the first woman's mind, with her history of infertility.

SOME MYTHS AND FACTS ABOUT MISCARRIAGE

In Ancient Greece, women were thought to miscarry if they were frightened by a clap of thunder. Fifty years ago psychologists attributed miscarriage to fear of pregnancy, neurosis and relationship difficulties. Many people still believe that a miscarriage results from strenuous physical activity. Or emotional shock. Or having sexual intercourse. While many women can remember a recent traumatic event, it is unlikely to have been the cause of the miscarriage.

The fact is that evidence indicates definite medical reasons for most miscarriages. Sometimes these medical reasons may seen unclear but even the vaguest medical explanation is more legitimate than myths about foods, temperatures, sexual activity and your own individual emotional lability.

The timing of the miscarriage provides a clue to the cause.

75% of miscarriages occur in the first twelve weeks. About half of these so-called 'early' miscarriages are due to abnormality in the embryo, or in the process of implantation in the woman's uterus. These abnormalities may be related to genetics or a chance mutation which has occured during fertilization or in the early growth of the embryo.

In what are called 'late' miscarriages, those that occur from the thirteenth to the twentieth week, the fetus is usually normal. However, there may be problems in its attachment to the placenta or to the uterus. There may also be abnormalities in the structure of the uterus, for instance, a double uterus. Sometimes the cervix is weak – and known by the unfortunate medical term, 'incompetent' – and dilates too early.

If a woman becomes seriously ill or contracts an infection, or suffers from malnutrition during the pregnancy, she may have an early or late miscarriage.

There is some evidence that the risk of miscarriage increases as a woman gets older.

It is probably true to say that in most cases, whether the miscarriage is early or late, the woman is shocked by the actual process. Few women expect a miscarriage to happen, so when it does, they are overwhelmed by the intensity of the physical and emotional process. Again, each woman is unique, so that her experience is different from every other woman's experience. There is considerable variation in the amount of pain and bleeding and in the time it takes for the miscarriage to be completed.

Most women who have experienced a miscarriage report that the actual event was very different from anything they might have anticipated.

Not only do women differ radically from one another in their reactions to miscarriage, but sometimes one woman with a history of miscarriage may respond differently each time it happens. Interestingly, women who have experienced several miscarriages sometimes tell of a series of similar, yet different, responses to the event.

Stella, a 32 year old counsellor has had four miscarriages at 10, 7, 17 and 12 weeks. She says,

'With the first miscarriage I was confused and very depressed. After the second miscarriage I was more sad and disappointed. I can only say that after the third miscarriage all my confidence was gone and I experienced the most awful shock to my whole system, both physically and psychologically. I become severely depressed after that miscarriage. I felt cheated, let down and very angry. Immediately after my fourth one, I felt sad, but relieved, because I had had such a terrible time, being so sick, that I knew instinctively that something was wrong. So at first, I was relieved, but that gave way to a feeling of total numbness. It was a long time before I could consider another pregnancy.'

Stella's responses tell of her confusion, disappointment and depression, all mixed with a sort of ambivalence, at least for some time. It's hard to make sense of an event like miscarriage. Many women continue to ask themselves, 'why did it happen?' And some become anxious about their future pregnancies and ability to carry the baby to full term. It is only natural to assume that knowing the cause of the first miscarriage might help to indicate whether future pregnancies could be at risk.

WHY DID IT HAPPEN?

When an explanation can be given to a woman she may find it helpful and empowering. However, for some women an explanation might still lead to concern and the question: 'Yes, but what caused the cause?'

If an explanation can't be given, then women report feeling adrift. They don't feel secure and believe their bodies have let them down. They begin to distrust themselves. Feeling self-blame, these women begin to feel guilty.

HERE'S A PRACTICAL SUGGESTION

The need for discussion with medical and nursing staff and emotional support from trusted friends and family is paramount for the woman. Articulate your need to people around you. It takes courage, but say: *'I need to talk about what happened. Will you let me talk about it?'* It's not easy, but you can do it. Don't allow people around you to depersonalize the event – miscarriage is a very personal experience.

When a woman is emotional and confused, it is important to let her talk about her 'baby' – not 'the foetus'. Her feelings need to be encouraged and brought out into the open.

If a woman is not permitted – or doesn't permit herself to talk about her emotions, her sense of guilt and confusion is compounded.

Remember that a woman begins to bond with her baby early in her pregnancy, so her feelings of loss are deep and intense.

Elizabeth Stein, in an article titled *Pregnant Pause*, shares her experience of miscarriage and then her experience of being pregnant and discovering there is something wrong with the baby inside her. She writes,

> 'Before my healthy baby was born three years ago, I had several miscarriages which caused intense grief. From the moment each pregnancy test returned positive, I started to dream. I would stand under the shower and talk to the baby. And every time I miscarried it was as traumatic as ending a relationship. Suddenly I was alone again, with a gnawing feeling that I would never hold my child in my arms.
>
> However, nothing could really prepare me for the experience of discovering,

halfway through my pregnancy, that the baby had a major foetal abnormality and would have to be terminated. At 17.5 weeks it wasn't just a surgical procedure. When there is a serious problem after 16 weeks, the birth must be induced and the mother admitted to hospital where she undergoes a minilabour that can take between 15 and 20 hours. I had no reason to believe there was anything wrong. I was in my late thirties but I'd had a chorionic villus sampling for chromosomal defects and been assured that my baby was fine. I had also been told I was carrying a boy and I had decided to name him Rafael.

I was feeling particularly sunny the day I clambered onto the bed for a routine ultrasound. I remember smiling as the nurse informed me about every stage of the examination. "The heart is beating strongly," she said, "Here's the baby's head, there are his arms and..."

"Is there something wrong?" I asked, but she brushed me off before disappearing to find the doctor.'

What Elizabeth Stein was to learn was shattering. Rafael had Potter Syndrome type 2A and meant that he could not survive outside the womb. She had to go through labour to deliver her son. A son she would never take home. After she got the news she describes her intense feelings: *'Weak-kneed, trembling and almost incoherent, I felt as though I'd been in an accident.'*

That fateful day when Elizabeth was given the news was the beginning of a journey for her which would end in a valuable lesson in life. She writes,

'The hospital's social workers had offered the service of a funeral director but I'm Jewish and, under our law, life only starts when the baby has taken his first breath. So Rafael couldn't have a Jewish funeral. Instead, my rabbi and I prayed for him and I dedicated a prayer book in his name and brought trees for him to be planted in Israel. It seemed to help.

'Almost six years have passed since I lost Rafael. It took me nearly two years to become pregnant again (I think it was all the emotional trauma) and there was one more early miscarriage. This time it was a blighted ovum (the pregnancy had failed to develop inside the womb) and once again I felt knocked over by a tidal wave of grief. However, just a couple of months later I was pregnant again and this time it was for keeps. I now have a healthy and

> *beautiful son who is just over three years old.*
> *Looking back, losing Rafael was certainly the most difficult experience I have faced, but it taught me about my inner strength. And most of all, it taught me how much to value the gift of life.'*

Like Elizabeth Stein, many women face the most difficult experience of a stillbirth. Again, many women search for a cause. And again, there is the need for medical and nursing staff as well as friends and relatives to be sensitive to the woman's feelings of vulnerability.

'TIME SEEMED TO STOP...'

These words are Melanie's. Melanie was 26 and expecting her first child. She discovered when she was 36 weeks pregnant that her baby had died. When she was told, she remembered not being able to say a word, as if she was paralysed. She says,

> *'Time seemed to stop. I didn't seem able to move. I couldn't say anything. But I was thinking, 'how am I going to tell my mum?' I had to go home and I kept wondering how I could spend the night at home with a dead baby inside me. I thought how cruel it was to go through labour for a dead baby. I don't think I slept much that night. My husband didn't know what to say. He hugged me and tried to console me physically, but I don't blame him for not saying anything – I mean what is there to say?*
>
> *'I didn't cry that night. I was too shocked. The next morning they started induction. I remember thinking I wanted a caesarean, just to get rid of the pain and get the baby out. I wanted to be detached from my dead baby, and I wanted to stop the emotional pain. But, really, I was glad I went through the birth because now I can remember it was a birth. I can now remember my baby girl and that she existed. Her name was Kerri-Anne.'*

Melanie naming her daughter means her baby can live on in her mind. It is an important ritual, signifying the existence, if only for a short time, of a child, with whom a mother has already bonded. Kerri-Anne's death was the end of the physical bond, but Melanie's emotional bond with her baby is memorialized.

In the past, stillborn babies were kept hidden from their parents. Mothers were either under anesthesia or covered with a drape to hide them from any view of the baby as he or she was being born. This practice was based on the belief that seeing a dead infant would leave a negative imprint on the mother's mind and cause her even more grief. It's probably also true to say that this practice shielded medical and nursing staff from facing their own anxieties concerning stillbirth.

Today a more enlightened and compassionate approach is used. It is now believed that seeing and holding the baby helps the mother – and father – face the reality of what has happened and helps begin the normal mourning process.

CIRCLE THIS

It is now considered to be important for a mother to spend time with her baby. She should be encouraged to look at her baby, to examine the baby's features, give him or her a name. Some mothers have a memento in the form of a photo of the baby – to remember their baby forever. Having a funeral or a ceremony, as in Elizabeth Stein's story, is also important. It is easier for a mother to mourn and to resolve her grief when the baby is a known person, not just a fantasy.

Although seeing the baby is a relief for many mothers, not all mothers want to see the baby.

Take note: The decision to see the baby should be left to the mother – and the parents – and the staff should support whatever decision they make. It is common practice to ask those parents who did not at first want to see the baby later in the day if they have changed their minds. At this point, the mother or the parents may decide to see the baby – or alternatively refuse as before. Because parents may ask many months later what their baby looked like, a picture can be taken for the baby's file and this picture can be offered to the parents if they ask.

Coming to terms with the mysterious paradox of stillbirth is difficult. Stillbirth confronts a mother with death preceding life. Her delivery is an ending. And her baby, who moved for months inside her is now outside – and forever still.

NO EXPLANATIONS

There are a number of babies who die despite having no malformations or other obvious pregnancy complications. These babies typically die in the last few weeks of the pregnancy.

Again the loss is unfathomable. Yet the desire to understand what had happened can never be satisfied in some cases. This can leave a woman anxious and uncertain about future children.

Stillbirth has been described as an 'empty tragedy'. After a stillbirth, the mother has a double sense of loss. Where there was a fullness, there is now a void.

CIRCLE THIS

You may recall how a mother, even with a live birth, may feel a sense of loss. Yet a mother with a baby, having lost her 'inside baby' has the consolation of her 'outside baby'. Some mothers may experience a puzzling and bewildering sadness to which they eventually adjust. However, with a stillbirth, a mother has to cope with not only the inner void, but an outer void as well.

FACING AN EMPTY NURSERY

Going home from the hospital empty-handed reinforces the reality of the mother's outer void. Eleni's baby son was stillborn. At the very end of her pregnancy she could no longer feel the baby's movements. When she was monitored, no heartbeat could be found. Eleni describes the desolation and panic she felt when she realised she would have to give birth to a dead baby. She says,

> *'My baby was born at 1.14 am. He was taken away and dressed and brought back to us. We were allowed to be alone with him. I thought he was the most beautiful baby I have ever seen. My love for him was overwhelming. My husband was very loving towards me and I could see he loved our baby. I could have held my baby all night. He looked perfect, just as if he was asleep. I was told he had died of placental insufficiency, the placenta was too small. It probably happened over the last weeks of pregnancy. The placenta apparently had deteriorated slowly so that he got less oxygen and food and got*

weaker and weaker. We were assured he finally 'went to sleep'. When he was finally taken away, I can't tell you how bewildered and empty I felt. Why did this happen to us? Why couldn't we take our baby home with us?'

For women like Eleni, facing an empty nursery is very painful. Some women have to face not only an empty nursery, but also the curiosity of their other children.

The empty nursery will be a constant reminder of your baby's absence. You may feel teary when you pack the baby clothes, blankets and shower gifts. Your milk-filled breasts will not only be physically painful, but will also remind you that you will not be mothering your baby.

Children at home may ask innocent questions. You may find yourself answering their questions repeatedly, 'I thought we were going to get a baby' and 'Why did our baby die?'

The outer void mentioned earlier, and the unanswerable questions also happen when a newborn baby dies.

Some babies will be alive at birth, but be critically ill. The mother will never take the baby home to the nursery. For the days, weeks or even months that ill babies live, the mother – and father – are tormented by feelings of confusion, uncertainty, hopes and fears. The biggest uncertainty is not knowing whether the baby will live or die.

In recent years, medical techniques have meant that more premature babies will survive. Nevertheless, the waiting, hoping and fearing is very stressful for the parents concerned. One woman, Nancy, whose son was born with spina bifida (a congenital defect of the spine which allows the spinal membranes (with or without cord tissue to protrude), had six weeks with him before he died. She says,

'I jumped at the chance of nursing my son – I didn't think they would let me. I was so depressed because the nurses were doing everything and I felt so inadequate. But when I nursed him, I began to feel like I was really his mother.'

Nancy and her husband felt supported by the hospital team and felt at ease with them. They were also grateful that the six weeks they had with their son gave them a chance to get to know him and to prepare themselves for his death. Nancy confides, *'I cherished those six weeks.'*

Having some memories to cherish is important in the face of such loss. Being able to survive such loss is a challenge.

SUDDEN INFANT DEATH SYNDROME

More than 15,000 parents a year survive 'crib death' or Sudden Infant Death Syndrome (SIDS). Even though research is intense and ongoing, crib death is baffling, because the cause or causes are still unknown.

Researchers have found that there are three themes that arise in the conversations with mothers whose babies have died suddenly – and seemingly inexplicably. These themes are:

1. Attachment to the baby

Unlike miscarriage and baby death due to illness or accident, the SIDS baby is most often at home where the baby has been nurtured and looked after. The peak time for babies lost to SIDS is between two to four months of age. In this time, the mother has bonded with and attached to her baby as a distinct individual with a unique personality. Because the death comes with no warning, there is sometimes a tendency to deny the baby has died. Some mothers continue to clean and rearrange the nursery, tend to the baby's clothes and maybe even prepare the formula. The baby may frequently be the subject of dreams. Dreams in which the mother is searching for, or caring for or playing with the baby.

2. Perception of the baby as healthy

At first, there is utter shock and disbelief that your healthy, happy baby was suddenly found dead. There had been no indicators of anything being wrong. The baby had never needed tests nor had the mother and father ever believed their baby's life was in danger. For instance, the day before, or even hours before your baby was being put to bed everything seemed normal. The baby's expression and movements were 'normal'. There was no indication of internal problems. The baby didn't cry or make any sound that indicated discomfort. The baby had been quietly sleeping in his or her familiar crib and never awakened. Many parents attempt to pinpoint an 'indicator' they think they might have overlooked. This leads to feelings of guilt.

3. The guilt factor

Many parents blame themselves immediately – and it's only natural given the mysterious circumstances of the baby's death. The beginnings of self-accusation are assisted by the process the parents must go through. Within hours of the baby's death, the parents are required to answer questions aimed to help make a diagnosis.

The guilt can escalate with parents extending the interrogation. When the legally required inquiry is complete, many parents continue to put themsleves through a silent grilling, still searching for a cause. Many mothers later report that they become obsessed with the logic that something or someone must be responsible. They feel compelled to identify a reason for the baby's death, no matter how implausible it may be.

A mother leaves no stone unturned. She considers everything she did prior to the baby's death: the clothing of the baby, the way the crib was prepared, the temperature of the room, what the baby had to eat. Did she miss a cry, a whimper, a sign something was wrong? She may recall, on reflection, a sound or gesture that she decides was a signal of the baby's distress, when in fact, it is a product of her own desperate imagination.

There are benefits of an autopsy. It provides a process which helps the mother and father discover that their fears have no factual basis. Discussing the autopsy report with a doctor, the parents will find that their real or imagined carelessness was not the reason for the baby's death.

An overwhelming finding in research and clinical practice is how life changes for most couples after a baby dies of SIDS. People are jolted into looking deeper at their lives, their ideas and their feelings after such a tragedy. One woman whose only child died of SIDS said, 'For the first time I truly understand how people feel who can't have children.' Other women say they are less selfish and more empathic with other people.

Carolyn Szybist wrote the following thoughts after her three month old son died of SIDS:

'I am a different person from the young woman I was just before my child died. I don't feel changed in a radical sense, but I am changed. It's sometimes difficult to relate to that person: to the youth, invincibility, and near simplicity. Sometimes I have difficulty remembering that young woman who was the mother of two children... It was a good time, laced with all the happiness and minor dissensions that are part of living.
And in one hellish moment, all of that changed. Changed as swiftly as if a bomb had been dropped into the core of our lives. Changed on a bright, sunny summer morning when I picked up the rigid, lifeless, distorted body of our young son.'

WHAT YOU CAN DO

Professionals in hospitals are able to provide contacts with other families and support groups for parents. Carolyn Szybist organised a support group and found she could come to terms with her tragedy. She saw a magazine article and that lead her to contact other people with experiences similar to her own. She found talking to these people, who had all been through their own unique tragedies, she could unlock long hidden feelings about her own tragedy. This happened three years after the event. Carolyn Szybist writes,

'... the release inside of me of so many locked up feelings can only be described as nearly exhilarating. It was a strange blend of hearing other people say what I had been feeling, and feeling along with them what I was hearing them say. When we all finally met as a group, it can only be described as a warm reunion of very old friends.'

This feeling that Carolyn Szybist so clearly articulates – that only someone who has been through a similar experience can truly understand – has made support groups an important part of many parents' lives. Support groups provide a sense of a collective – and can help parents overcome the terrible isolation they feel in their personal grief.

Take note:
- As a mother, you may be overcome by grief and sadness, but remember, don't neglect your partner's feelings. He has lost a child too.

- Other family members, including children should be part of the process of detachment from the baby. Seeing and touching a dead sibling will not damage a child, as long as she or he is properly prepared (and there is no gross abnormality of the baby). A child's imagination is more likely to be frightening than being introduced to the reality of death. If a child is excluded, they might develop fantasies which can become problematic.

HOW YOU CAN HELP OTHERS

If you know someone who has experienced miscarriage, stillbirth or whose baby has died of crib death, allow her to talk about her feelings. Acknowledge her loss by sending a card or making a sympathetic remark. Don't remain silent. Remember to be particularly sensitive around the time the child was to be born, or on the anniversary of the baby's death. Remember, the woman is not alone. Include her partner and the rest of the family in your consideration.

If you've experienced the loss of a child, consider all the previous comments made by women and find yourself a support group. The self-help checklist below summarizes some important issues:

SELF-HELP CHECKLIST

- Acknowledge your grief, even if others don't understand. You have lost a child and that is a tragedy. You have every right to grieve
- Try to view and touch your baby, if possible
- Acknowledge your child's individuality and unique personhood. Give the child a name and a memorial service or funeral
- Be aware that your partner and family are also grieving
- Find out as much as you can about your loss. Listen to professionals. Read pamphlets and books to help dispel the mystery that can add to your grief and depression.

8

VULNERABLE POINTS AND PROCESSES

*It is the image in the mind that binds us to our
lost treasures, but it is the loss that shapes the image.*

COLETTE

We all need to find our own rhythms to live by. This will be a constant search for there is no one pattern that will work for a whole lifetime. And there will always be some points and processes in our lives that may make us vulnerable. Part of the rhythm by which many of us like to live is embodied in the theme of 'mastery' over life – a sense of control. Dr Lynn P. Rehm, professor of psychology at the University of Houston has said, *'Particularly relevant to depression is people's sense of control over their lives – their ability to do what they want and to get what they want out of life.'*

However, there are times when a sense of control is not available to us. A sense of control can be gained by having choices. Often our choices are limited in reality, or in our perception. But finding choices and acting on them helps to make us feel less vulnerable. It allows us to believe we are taking responsibility for ourselves and our lives.

Remember, it is important to assert your right to choose whenever possible. By doing so, you'll feel less vulnerable.

Vulnerable points in a woman's life relate to experiences at particular life stages or crisis situations which undermine the woman's self-image and increase her vulnerability to depression. They take away a woman's sense of control. Some of these points and processes may relate to the motherhood role and the dual role of mother and paid worker. Other points and processes may involve depression resulting from locked emotions following adoption and losing your parent or spouse and the psychosocial crisis experienced in the aftermath of an affair.

All these points and processes will be discussed in this chapter.

One vulnerable point in a woman's life was touched on earlier. It is motherhood, and the process by which a woman takes on a nurturing role.

Erma Bombeck in her amusing book, **Motherhood: The Second Oldest Profession**, writes, *'One of the biggest complaints about motherhood is the lack of training... Motherhood is an art. And it is naive to send a mother into an arena for twenty years with a child and expect her to come out on top.'*

VULNERABLE POINT 1: JUGGLING ACTS AND OTHER PERFORMANCES

Callie suggests the following job description . . .

Occupation: Mother
Job description: Chief cook, bottle washer, first-aid nurse, floor scrubber, nappy washer, budget-controller, peace-maker, comforter-in-chief, moral minder
Hours of employment: Endless

Before Callie, a 30 year old stay-at-home mother of two young children, became a mother, she was a personal assistant. She says:

> *'Don't get me wrong. I love the kids. I'd die if anything happened to either of them. But I detest being a mother. I feel like I've been duped. No-one told me there'd be rotten sides to motherhood. And it didn't occur to me. But now, I know. My life has changed and I've lost all my freedom. It's freedom of all sorts – financial, physical and emotional. I don't get paid for the huge responsibilites I have, I can't be my own person because I'm constantly in fear – and guilt – about putting my needs ahead of the children's.'*

Many women come to motherhood completely unaware of its drawbacks. Then they discover them and often they feel they are lacking as mothers. Instead of seeing the situation for what it is – a difficult, full-time task which demands enormous personal resources, these women find themselves deficient.

Motherhood is a demanding business. It's 24 hours a day, seven days a week and there are no days off from the doubt, worry and concern. It's endless.

There is often a huge gap between myth and reality. Even today, mothers are depicted in television commercials as young, cheerful and energetic. That's the myth. Then there's the reality.

Dr E. James Lierberman, a psychiatrist who in the 1970s reported on the future of the American family commented: *'Child-rearing is the most difficult task that most ordinary mortals will ever undertake.'*

While it is true that in today's world more and more fathers are becoming involved in actively raising their children, the bulk of the responsibility still falls on the woman as wife and mother.

Many years ago, Dr Kalra Tulsky in **The Health of the Housewife**, defined mental health as 'a balance of frustrations and gratifications'. For some women, this definition rings true for motherhood – that state which is about frustrations and gratifications. Sometimes the gratifications outweigh the frustrations and at other times, that situation is reversed. But, for those women who find they experience more frustrations than gratifications, the experience of motherhood is riddled with dilemmas.

Although women today certainly have many more choices than their mothers and infinitely more choices than their grandmothers, some basic expectations and ideas are enduring. One is that the role of mother is a highly valued one. Above all, it must not be compromised. Therein lies the difficulty for some women.

In **The Motherhood Myth**, Shirley Radl examines motherhood and the driving ideology behind it. She says:

'Motherhood, then, is both a career and an affliction. It has caused many women to seek nothing beyond, caused many others to stifle their creative

spirits and their dreams for a career of a different order, and caused still others to wear themselves out trying to do justice to two careers'.

Selwa, 44, who recently returned to work after 14 years of being a stay-at-home wife and mother, refers to these 14 years as her 'menial mother' years. She laughs about her frustrations and depression during those years. But her laugh sounds hollow and as she speaks there is the impression that she's yet to accept those years of her life as valuable. There is a sense in which she felt invalidated in her role as mother, and in turn, she has invalidated her experience. She says:

'I knew I'd made a mistake shortly after my first child was born. I'd been a legal secretary and I enjoyed my work, but then I got married and pregnant before I had really thought it all through. There was a lot of pressure from both my family and my husband's to 'do the right thing' and stay at home with the children.

'I had two and although my husband wanted more, I didn't. I've always hated that motherhood and apple-pie image, and before long, I found myself trapped in it! I was expected to be the dutiful wife and good mother. It's funny how people can change.

'My husband was always supportive and I felt I could be my own person, but as soon as I became a mother, he started to redefine me – as his wife and my child's mother. It was so stereotypical – suddenly I was transformed from career-woman to the woman's magazine ideal of motherhood. And I hated it.

'I hated it for fourteen years, but in a strange way, I also felt guilty and I couldn't return to work until both kids were less dependent on me. I see my menial mother years as lost years and I spent a good part of that time unhappy and depressed. I felt I'd lost some of myself.'

Selwa's sentiments were echoed by Pauline. She also believes she's lost some of her life to 'the menial mother years' and was depressed most of the time she was at home looking after her four children.

Pauline is 59 and remembers the days when women were only depicted as being happy when they'd discovered a new washing powder. She comments:

'In my time, the commercials were so insulting to women. Detergents, baby powder and baby food commercials made motherhood seem like the ultimate act of creativity and gracious living. Judging from those commercials, the most serious decision a woman and mother had to make was which brand of peanut butter to feed her family or which washing powder to get the clothes whiter than white.

'I hated those years of being at home, being expected to be at home – because women didn't work – not routinely like they do today. My husband would have been horrified if I'd gone out to work. It was a matter of pride – the male breadwinner and all that. Thank goodness things have changed today. I envy the young women of today. They have so much more choice and freedom.

'I didn't mind looking after the children – there were four of them – but I did resent the loneliness – I craved for adult company – but young mothers didn't network like they do today. I lived a life of boredom, doing boring tasks and feeling low most of the time.'

It's easy to understand how Pauline felt depressed with her lot. She was being sold a product – motherhood – which didn't live up to its promises for her. The constant companionship of small children can be annoying and stifling. Some women crave intellectual stimulation, or even the company of other adults. Being a mother can be isolating and depressing in its never-ending demands. Pauline is probably right when she says that young women of today have different expectations and greater opportunities. What's more, advertising agencies are no longer selling the big myths – some might prefer to call them lies – that they did in Pauline's day.

However, even today, women who stay at home with their children need others around them to value their choice. These women need to be seen as intelligent, capable people.

In the book ***Tea and Tranquillizers***, mentioned in a previous chapter, the heroine continues her diary entry with:

'Monday 15th. Saw a child expert on TV this evening. She'd been blessed with a TV interview because of her startling revelation that women were missing out on the stimulating creative business of child raising by returning to

interesting well-paid jobs.

'*I used to believe that kind of thing... I remember when I had a job, before I had the children, how I looked down on housewife friends who complained of being miserable and unhappy at home. I thought they were apathetic and ignorant. I thought they were expressing views that were fashionable rather than true. I really thought I'd be happy making dragons out of empty egg boxes all day. I really thought children were interested in dragons made of empty egg boxes.*

'*No-one really told me what being a wife and mother meant. I think that's wrong. I shall tell younger women the truth, if I'm ever asked. But will they believe me in the face of all those ads? They'll think me apathetic, ignorant and that I'm expressing views fashionable rather than true.*'

THE HASSLE OF HOUSEWORK

Housework is work. But it's work with little status attached to it. It is done for love or because of emotional and financial ties.

Housework generally is understood to include things like shopping, cooking, cleaning, washing clothes and tidying, caring for children and other dependants and all the other miscellaneous tasks associated with running a house on a daily basis. All this means that the woman serves others and this leads to sex role and power conflicts. Even when the woman has a paid job, she is still expected to perform most of the housework duties. Recent studies show that women are continuing to carry most of the burden for domestic labor. This leads to a situation where some women are sharing economic responsibilities with their husbands, but on the domestic front, they're on their own.

The way we look at housework is interesting. Mostly, people still see is as non-work. Because it's unpaid, it's not work. Strange logic, but true.

Lesley, 31, does casual work on a check-out counter. She sees her main role as homemaker, as does her husband. She comments:

'*It really annoys me when Jay tells me I'm a free agent. He says I complain too much and I don't know I'm onto a good thing. Yeah I say to him – cooking, cleaning and washing your dirty underwear – great one. He says I can do things in my own time without any pressure from anybody. He just doesn't understand. Is he kidding? No pressure? I'm under a ton of pressure all the time. I'd like to see how he'd react if I didn't feel any pressure and did the laundry in my own time!'*

This idea that housework is a set of easy tasks with no boss and no set hours leads to the sort of thinking which says housework isn't 'really' work. Ann Oakley, the British sociologist, in her book **Housewife**, reveals that there are enormous pressures for some women to do their housework impeccably. She found that husbands are often critical of housekeeping standards. Some women get depressed about their housekeeping lot.

Oakley found that for many working-class women, with fewer choices regarding paid work and even fewer choices in terms of paid help, housework is no better than work in a factory. For these women housework meant a daily grind of cold houses and apartments, little money, screaming children and few pieces of household equipment – all guaranteed to make life difficult for the woman. Oakley found that cooking and shopping were the most popular tasks, the first because it can be creative and the second because it offers a chance to get out of the house. Considerable dissatisfaction was expressed by the women regarding their housework tasks. One woman from the Oakley study said: *'When I was working I used to get a tremendous kick out of doing... housework. But now I'm doing it every day it really is the biggest bore of my life.'*

Diane Harpwood's heroine writes in her diary about her average day. Her diary entry captures the tedium of housework:

> *'Wednesday 3rd. Took Lucy to school, came home, had a cuppa with Katie, did the washing, made the beds and tidied the house, fetched Lucy home from school, cooked tea, washed up, took the children to bed, read them a story, tidied the toys away, washed up after David's meal, sat down at eight, made supper at ten and now I've come to bed, ten-fifteen.*
> *Thursday 4th. Ditto except substitute ironing for washing.'*

Many women report feeling like they are 'small-minded' when they are housebound and doing housework on a daily basis. One woman told me that there's a certain feeling of unreality about life as a homemaker and mother. She said women like her 'live in our own little world'.

Certainly times are changing. More men are now more willing to help with little household tasks. Recent research has highlighted that men like doing the shopping, vacuuming and house-maintenance tasks the best. But the fact remains: few men regard the housework as their responsibility.

Kim 28, a stay-at-home mother has found a remedy to her feelings of frustration and depression about her husband not appreciating her efforts. She's discovered the power of sex as barter. She says:

> *'I hate being taken for granted. I've got two small kids and a husband who expects to be waited on hand and foot. I got very down about all of it some time ago. I went to see my doctor and he tried to put me on tranquillisers. I told him I needed more understanding. I can't believe some men. They think that the moment you find a bit of spunk, you've lost your mind. I didn't need settling down with pills, I needed to take action.*
>
> *'I talked to a friend and we came up with this brilliant idea. We'd withhold sex from our husbands until things changed. I knew my husband would sulk and then he'd go into withdrawals and then I'd have him. It was a great plan – and it worked! I've never felt better about things. He pays much more attention to me, the kids and what I go through every day. He'd better or I'll starve him again!'*

Sex as barter. Sex as weapon. It seems it might be a commodity that the desperate, depressed homemaker can use to her advantage.

Housework then is work. It is time-consuming and can be very exhausting. It can lead to 'happy homes' or to conflict and contradictions. Society's gender division of labor is still very embedded in housework.

A FINAL NOTE ON MOTHERHOOD

Everyone knows what a mother is. She's the one who gives you aspirin when you have a cold and reads you stories before bed. She's the one who makes you wear galoshes when it's raining. But, neither love nor sudsier suds can make some mothers like the endless responsibility, boredom and drudgery that all mothers know deep down go with caring for children and running a home.

In an article titled *The hardest job in the world* in *Ladies' Home Journal*, Mary Kay Berger said *'Nobody prepares you for what it's like'*. Her stay-at-home mum's job was vastly different from her previous busy executive life. However, she concludes, that there are rewards – and four little words play a large part in meeting a mom's needs for recognition. Mary Kay says, *'You don't see immediate results with this kind of work. But when one of your kids says, 'Mommy, I love you,' it keeps you going'.*

WHAT YOU CAN DO

Feeling that you don't deserve attention, or at least, that your family comes first, can be dangerous to your mental health in the long-term. You can only suppress your needs for so long!

When you're feeling vulnerable and you're down in the dumps, it's hard to say, 'my needs are important'. And you may feel guilty when you do. But, if you deny your needs, they have a way of coming to the surface, and oozing out of the cracks, sooner or later – and often when you least expect it!

Remember, in an earlier chapter, you practised being assertive. Now's the time to do so again.

Exercise

Say 'my needs are important' to yourself
Acknowledge that you as a person are important.
You do not deserve to feel vulnerable and depressed.
You deserve to get help if you need it.
Having given to your family for so long, now is the time you need something for yourself.

Practise your affirmation: 'My needs are important'
It's not a matter of being selfish, but if you don't get your needs met, then you won't be in a position to meet your family's needs. Remember how Callie shared her fear and guilt with us earlier in this chapter, about 'putting my needs ahead of the children's'? It's a common mistake to believe you're not being a good mother if you consider your own needs for one moment.

It's time to banish the fear and the guilt. If your needs aren't being met and you feel depressed and depleted, you won't have any energy or inclination left to meet your family's needs.

So practise your affirmation again: 'My needs are important'
Most importantly – you have to believe it!

So say it again: 'My needs are important'
If motherhood provides an oftentimes challenging – and sometimes depressing scenario for some women, what about the impact of dual roles on women's lives?

VULNERABLE POINT 2: THE TIGHT-ROPE BALANCING ACT

The role of women in society has radically changed in most western countries. Since the 1960s there has been a large increase in the number of women entering paid employment. In the U.S., in 1950, women constituted 30% of the labour force and by the early 1990s this had increased to 49%. The statistics tell a dramatic tale. One of the significant changes in the female labour force had been the influx of married working women, particularly in part-time jobs. Today, 70% of married females work and over 41% of women with children under five are in employment, compared with 24% in 1983.

In recent years, two-thirds of all women with children under 18 were in paid employment and the fastest growing segment of the workforce is working mothers with children under the age of three. In the past fifteen years, paid employment rates for women aged 18 to 44 years with new-born children rose from 18% to 51%.

While these facts and figures are intriguing in themselves, it is the consequences of the facts and figures which are even more interesting. What are the implications for women and their mental health – given the rates at which they are taking up dual roles of mother and paid worker?

For some women, the tight-rope balancing act of being a partner, parent and paid worker is simply a breeze. We all know women who manage it all, seemingly without any difficulties. On the other hand, we also know those women who have 'lost it', because the stresses and strains on them in occupying too many roles has come at the cost of their mental health. Marina is one such woman. Her three children are at school and Marina works full-time as a sales assistant, out of economic necessity. She says,

> *'If I had my way, I'd only work part-time. It gets me down having to rush around like I do. I keep telling myself I don't have to kill myself, but what's the alternative? Sometimes I don't sleep well worrying about things not being done. I feel guilty I can't do more. The kids help sometimes, but I try to spare them too much housework. I want them to get good grades, so I don't expect too much of them. I don't expect anything from my husband.'*

Guilt is something many women feel intensely, under their role strain. Learning to manage your guilt is the first step to preventing that downward depressive spiral from overtaking you.

The following exercise will help you understand what you are inclined to feel guilty about – and how you might begin to change the situation.

Exercise: Managing your guilt

What will you feel guilty about today? Here's a list of some of the things women feel guilty about. Be honest! Tick the ones you'd worry about:

I'd worry about this

1. The house is a mess. You invite a friend around. She's early. She arrives ten minutes after you get home. ☐
2. The breakfast dishes are still on the table. You see your friend looking at them. ☐
3. If you decided to get help you'd probably clean up before the cleaner arrived. ☐
4. If your child is experiencing problems at school, you suspect it's because you didn't give them quality time or because you should have read with them more. ☐
5. You never get a moment for yourself, because when you're at home, you never take a break from the children. ☐
6. You feel bad about taking some time off work because of the children. (eg. their sickness) ☐
7. Your ageing mother complains she's lonely and you feel it's your fault. ☐
8. If you work outside the home, you feel you're not a good wife because you're tired in the evenings. ☐

9. When things are left undone around the home, you feel guilty because you haven't done them. You consider it to be your job. ☐
10. Your husband asks you to type up his résumé and you know he's better at the keyboard than you. But you do it for him anyway. ☐

Look at your ticks. How did you go?

If you scored 0–2 ticks
You are a little anxious about life. What are the particular areas you ticked?
• Your children? • Your relationship? • Your parents? • Your work? • Your home?

If you scored 2 – 4 ticks
You've scored like the average guilty woman. You're guilty about the sorts of things that make women feel guilty. Why not change it?

If you scored 4 ticks or more
You have decidedly pronounced yourself guilty! You know you are vulnerable in particular areas and maybe others around you know you feel guilty. And maybe they are sometimes tempted to take advantage of you!

WAYS OF MANAGING YOUR GUILT

First, you must decide not to feel guilty.
Secondly, you must decide you will not make yourself vulnerable.
Thirdly, you must act on it!

Practise saying: 'Would you like to help around the home because I'm tired?' to your older children and your husband.

Practise saying: 'Would you look after my children while I go out and play tennis?' to your mother, sister, friends, neighbours. And practice saying anything else that will help you get rid of your guilt!

Complete the following sentence: I know I give others my attention and lately I've been neglecting myself, so I'm going to…

And make sure you give yourself the attention you need and deserve! And no guilt allowed!

Choices about continuing in dual roles have to be made by each woman. For some women, the costs of continuing to 'do it all' might mean feeling de-energised and depressed. For others, the tension involved in the dual roles can be managed – with care – because they know that to surrender the paid work role would almost certainly result in depression.

Yvonne, a lawyer is representative of this sort of woman. Before returning to legal practise full-time, she was beginning to feel depressed with the demands of being 'the perfect stay-at-home mum'. She says,

> *'Okay, it's stressful being all things to all people, but it's a lot more interesting and stimulating than being at home with the kids all day. I have the good fortune of having enough money to get help and not feel too guilty about family life.'*

There it is again – guilt. But as Yvonne suggests, those women who can afford to pay for outside help and support have an advantage. They can assuage their guilt, at least some of the time.

Trying to be Superwoman doesn't work for most of us. All it does is make us vulnerable – to feeling guilty and depressed.

Take note: Here are some things that might help . . .
1. Get help!
2. Make a list. This list will act to remind you of the 'fundamentals', the essential things that need to be done. This list could become your secret weapon!
3. Make a schedule and then keep to it. In this schedule give yourself one 'day off'. And then remember to take it!

Maybe you have other ideas on what might help you in your tight-rope balancing act. Here's your chance: *Write some ideas here:*

_____
_____
_____

At times, women become so depressed they can't see their way out. By reflecting and coming up with other possibilities, a sense of control begins to emerge. When this starts to happen, a woman can begin to see the reality – and often, the hidden humour – in the tensions of her tight-rope balancing act. Here's an excercise to help you gain control:

| Exercise | Delegating to others |

Write down a list of the jobs you expect yourself to do.

_____
_____
_____
_____

How many of these jobs would you like to delegate?

_____
_____
_____
_____

Why are you still doing them? Write your excuses here!

_____
_____
_____
_____

HARD LUCK STORIES

Clinging to our hard luck stories is a good way of assuring a sense of powerlessness. Beating yourself up because you're not perfect – you can't be what Yvonne calls, 'all things to all people' is not an empowering strategy. In fact, it guarantees to take away your sense of control.

We all have external pressures on us. However, it is sometimes the internal pressures or 'drivers' that tip the balance. It is these internal drivers, these additional pressures we put on ourselves at work and at home that can push us into a downward spiral. What are some of the things that drive us?

Drivers are:

Be perfect – Be good, do everything, never make a mistake.

I want to please you – Women learn this early. It is part of our 'nurturing' training.

Hurry up – Often this is learned early in life. It can become a driver making us feel we have to achieve everything in the fastest, possible time. Never mind the quality, just watch the speed!

Try hard – This is another early lesson which can become a driver demanding that you put 110% into everything.

Be strong – This early message can become a driver when you feel you need to achieve everything in a day, even if you're exhausted by the end of it.

These drivers can help you achieve, but they can also be your undoing emotionally. These drivers can become 'overdrivers'. It is when a woman finds herself telling a hard luck story and realizing she is overdoing things that the negative effect of drivers is felt. I've known women to become depressed because they concentrate intensely on 'being perfect' and doing things perfectly – all to the exclusion of things that actually need to be done.

Being perfect – wanting everything to go well has sometimes meant women being vulnerable to suggestions and options which may return to haunt them. One traumatic life event which leads to depression immediately, and often chronically over a lifetime, is giving up your baby for adoption.

Hundreds of thousands of women in the United States, Britain and Australia have surrendered babies for adoption. Interviews with them, many years later, reveal that at the time they relinquished their babies, they experienced depression, isolation and a sense of relational disconnection Even years later, these emotions continue to reverberate through the women's lives.

VULNERABLE LIFE POINT 3: GIVING UP A CHILD

'I ONLY WANTED THE BEST FOR HER'

These are the words of Jeanette, now 46. She relinquished her daughter, whom she called Rose, 27 years ago. At 24, Jeanette married and subsequently had two children. She and her husband are still together. Over the years, Jeanette suffered from chronic depression and was hospitalised on three separate occasions. She kept Rose a secret for the first ten years of her marriage. She feared her husband would not understand. She was right. He responded angrily, accusing her of not 'trusting' him by being honest with him about her past from the beginning. Jeanette remembers that this encounter triggered a moderate depression in her. Jeanette tells me she still believes she did 'the right thing', yet at times, she has doubts and recriminations.

The phenomenon of adoption creates a triangle, sometimes called the 'adoption triad'. Three lives merge, diverge and often merge many years down the track. There are always at least three players: a birth mother, a child and adoptive parents. In the past, the adoption process was secretive and 'closed'. It was thought 'for the best' that the players in the 'adoption triad' remain anonymous: the birth mother's identity was secret as was the adoptive parents' details. Many birth mothers report people telling them to 'forget' their child and 'to get on with life'. Young women were routinely told that if they really loved their child they would surrender it for adoption. While these sentiments were well-intentioned, they were seriously flawed.

Researchers have since learned that the majority of relinquishing mothers could not 'forget' their child. The pain, the depression and the unresolved grief – and guilt – became part of their lives. Many mothers have stumbled emotionally through the years, haunted by the knowledge that their child is living somewhere, with someone – but where and with whom? They hoped that the child was happy.

Today, the adoption process is open and even those mothers who relinquished their children years ago, may hope to have contact with their adult children – if both parties agree to that contact. For reunion to succeed, there has to be true desire to meet from both the point of view of the birth mother and the adult child.

In Jeanette's case, her wish was reciprocated and she met Rose, or rather Shannon, as her adoptive parents had called her. Jeanette says,

'I never forgot Rose. There have been times over the past 27 years when I've felt so guilty. I was hospitalised for depression several times. I felt bad, but I knew

> *I'd done the right thing really. How could I raise a child on my own? I only wanted the best for her. But you always have nagging doubts don't you? When I found I could contact her I was so happy, and nervous. I couldn't sleep the night before. At first, my husband didn't appreciate my need to meet my daughter. He said, 'You should leave it alone'. But I couldn't. I wanted to see her and I wanted to tell her I loved her.'*

Jeanette had hoped for a 'high' on reuniting with her daughter. In her case, her expectation was matched by reality. She continues,

> *'I've gained a lot out of meeting Rose, or Shannon. I've gained my baby back and I now know she's grown into a healthy, intelligent young woman. I don't have to wonder whether she's happy. I told her I loved her, and she said she loved me and we both cried. The hardest thing was accepting she belongs to another family and that there will always be gaps in our life together. We now see each other every few months and it's always good. We've become good friends. That's more than I hoped for. And I think she's starting to forgive me.'*

There's the guilt again – and the hope of forgiveness. Jeanette and Shannon are a success story. However, there are other results of adoption reunion which end in disappointment, or in people being 'found' only to be 'lost' again, after one or two contacts. Expectations can run high and reality has to work hard to keep up. Sometimes, the people involved in the adoption triad find themselves heading in directions they had not envisaged.

CIRCLE THIS

A reunion generates an emotional kaleidoscope. A sense of depression, after the 'high' of reunion, is not uncommon.

Why did my mother have me adopted at birth? This is a big question many adopted people ask of themselves – and many now proceed to ask their birth mother. Women may feel angry with their birth mother for having abandoned them. Women often have all sorts of fantasies about the circumstances of their birth, and some of these are confirmed. Others are found to be just that – fantasies and imaginings.

FINDING YOUR MOTHER

'Hello, mum, you don't know me...'

According to Marleen, these were the first words she said to her mother on the phone. Marleen, 32 said she'd thought little about her adoption until her teenage years when her relationship with her adoptive mother broke down.

Looking back, Marleen believes she was depressed, but no-one put that label on her feelings of malaise. At about the age of 16, she began wondering what it would be like to meet her birth mother. She'd been told she was adopted when she was 8, as had her 5 year old brother. Marleen had never felt she fitted in. She felt so different from her adoptive parents in looks, personality and even in sense of humour. Marleen was to spend another ten years thinking about her birth mother before she finally went to an agency which helped her establish contact. Her birth mother was traced and agreed to the contact. Marleen can still remember her jubilation when she was given permission to ring.

Marleen's reunion with her natural mother was a positive event. She says:

> *'I'll never forget the day I first laid eyes on my mother. Here was this woman who was an older version of me. When she hugged me I felt a warm sensation flood by body. We got on well from the start. She lives in another State, so we see each other when we can. We've established an easy relationship.'*

Yet, Marleen admits to feeling let down by her mother's reluctance to talk about the adoption itself, or the circumstances surrounding it. Her mother still finds it difficult to describe Marleen's father or the relationship she had with him. Marleen is disappointed her mother doesn't feel she can fill in these gaps for her. But Marleen remains hopeful.

Marleen's story shows how even a positive reunion can raise issues which can lead to a sense of disappointment.

Adopted children sometimes report that the truths they uncover turn out to be a lot more complicated than the dreams they had treasured for so long. Not knowing your genetic roots may be a contributing element to feeling not in control of your life. It's worthwhile considering reunion with your mother

– or with your child – but once the search is over, it's back to reality. Searching and finding generate expectations and anticipation, while the reunion has the potential to trigger an emotional kaleidoscope.

There will need to be an adjustment to a life which includes new information, perhaps more complex information, some gaps and maybe regrets and recriminations. And, of course there will be joy about the emotional reconnection.

Nevertheless, after the music swells, the players stroll off into the sunset and the picture fades... there is the new reality.

New realities challenge us to find a new sense of control. One new reality which plunges many women into a depression is the loss of a parent, particularly the loss of a mother, our same-sex parent.

VULNERABLE POINT 4: LOSING YOUR PARENT

'I felt paralysed, like parts of my body didn't work...'

You may recall Blythe in the first chapter saying how profoundly she'd been affected by her mother's death. She said:

> *'I've only been depressed really badly once. It was after my mother died. We had a very close relationship. The depression affected my whole body. I felt paralysed, like parts of my body didn't work. I had terrible indigestion, I couldn't think straight I was so distraught with the loss.'*

It's important to remember that surviving the loss of a parent is a major life event. Even if you are an adult when your parent dies, you respond to their death as the child of your parent. Common reactions to the death of a parent include guilt and anger, feeling vulnerable, knowing that you are closer to death because the buffer of one generation has gone, feeling like an orphan and frustration because you might have something more you wanted to say or do.

In a sense, no matter how old you are, you have lost something very fundamental – the relationship or the potential of relationship with your mother or father. Only a child – daughter or son – can fully understand everything the parent represents to them. Some women feel especially lost and this feeling is reflected by the metaphors they use.

For instance, one woman, Shirley, 44, said *'I lost my mother confessor, my home base where I always knew I'd be accepted'*. Another woman, Delvene, 31, said, *'My father was like an anchor in my life – physically, emotionally and spiritually'*. And Maggie, 57 said, *'I lost both my parents within three months of each other. I guess I've lost my home. The place I always knew I could retreat to.'*

Although you are aware that immortality is impossible, your subconscious mind may have nurtured the irrational belief that your parents' death may not actually occur. At one time or another, we all hold the belief that a parent can live forever. Even in the face of obvious challenge to this belief, our denial is deep and often entrenched. We don't want to face life without our parents in the background of our lives.

When you lose a parent, you may feel extraordinarily vulnerable to the world in general. This is echoed in comments like *'I feel like an orphan'*. The forsaken child in us all may feel this more intensely when a mother dies.

Women have reported feeling anxious about taking on new responsibilities and presiding over the younger generation. When a parent dies you begin to view yourself as the 'older generation'. As Shirley confides, *'I realised, with some trepidation, that I was the mummy now and forever'*.

CIRCLE THIS

It is a fact that losing a parent leaves a void in your life. When the parent-child relationship ends, there is a sense of discontinuity. Again, this is felt more keenly with the loss of the same-sex parent. Women often say things like, *'I wish my mother was here now to see me and be proud of me'* or *'to advise me what to do'*, or *'help me out now'*.

Women often tell of how empty and despairing they are, knowing that they can't just pick up the phone and call their mother. I know I felt this way – and I still do. I miss my mother's presence. I long for a day in town with her. I would like to enjoy her company. Longing, yet knowing it will never again be.

A woman may identify strongly with her own mother. This identification may be physical, mental, social, emotional or spiritual – or all of these. In losing your mother, you may want to reflect on similarities and likenesses that you want to treasure and remember. It may also be helpful to have an object to keep as a physical reminder of your mother. This object, which was your mother's personal effect, serves two functions for you: it is something you can cherish and it is visible proof of your mother's earthly life.

CIRCLE THIS

It is natural for you to want to hold, look at and own something tangible that represents your mother's individuality and former presence. If a woman can't find some memento to treasure, she may become despairing and distressed.

One client told me she became extremely distressed, almost hysterical, when she found that one of her mother's rings, which her mother had promised her, was given to her niece. She became depressed and we discussed how she must take control and do something about it. We spoke about her need to have something to hold onto – and something which she considered hers – and a reminder of her mother. Finally, she decided to write a letter to her niece, explaining her feelings and asking for the ring. The story ends well. Not only was she relieved for having written out her feelings, but the ring was sent to her almost immediately.

Allowing and expressing your feelings is crucial if you are to get over depression. It is the first step in taking control. Many women find counselling or therapy helps them release their feelings and work through their loss. One self-help strategy that helps many women is writing about their feelings.

You might like to try the following exercise – which guides you through writing about your loss.

Exercise Writing about your feelings

Take a piece of paper and your favorite pen and look at the following questions. Answer them as honestly as you can.

Your relationship with your parent
What kind of relationship did you have? What were the most important aspects of your relationship?

Your parent's perception of you
How would your parent have described your personality, character, appearance and capability? How is this similar to or different from the way you see yourself?

Your strongest emotional responses to your parent's death
Did you feel vulnerable? angry? afraid? despairing? relieved? Why do you think you responded as you did?

Your regrets
What more did you want to say or do? If your parent were still alive today, how would you take care of this unfinished business?

What specifically do you miss?
Do you miss knowing you can't call around on Sunday? Make that phone call twice a week? Share your parent's sense of humour? Talk over problems? Be offered advice – even if unsolicited?

Unfinished aspects of relationships can be tormenting. By reflecting on matters and writing them down, you can start to address unfinished business from both sides of the relationship. This notion of unfinished business is also raised by the death of a spouse or partner.

VULNERABLE LIFE POINT 5: LOSING YOUR SPOUSE

The death of a partner or spouse is one of the most stressful events that a person can experience. After a long relationship, a woman suffering the loss of her spouse can feel like the world has turned upside down. Everything suddenly seems unfamiliar and nothing makes sense. Being alone suddenly, after perhaps a lifetime of being half of a couple can be terrifying. A woman may experience life as empty and hopeless. There seems to be little point in going on alone. There seems little point in doing things, because there is no-one to share them with.

It's often thought to be the case that the closer and more intimate the relationship, the more devastating the loss will be. And the greater the potential for vulnerability. Readjustment after bereavement takes time. Often lots of time.

Losing a spouse can feel like losing an essential part of yourself. It can be painful and disorienting. You may not be sure of how to cope with life in general. Sometimes, you may not be sure you want to try to cope.

As one widow, Celia, 63 confides, 'I'm so tired all the time. Everything is too much effort. It's like part of me is missing.' Immediately after your loss you may experience depressed mood, tiredness, prolonged crying and insomnia. It's like sadness, exhaustion and despair pervade your life.

Again, there are individual differences. Your emotions will be influenced by your personality, the nature of your relationship, the duration of your relationship, the cause of your partner's death, your age, previous losses you've experienced and other factors.

However, there are some common feelings and concerns. The following statements reveal some of these feelings and concerns:

- I feel as if I've lost part of myself
- I feel as if I've lost my best friend
- I feel angry
- I feel afraid
- I feel guilty about something (or many things) I did
- I feel like I'm going through an identity crisis

Not everyone will identify with all of these statements, but some of them are probably familiar to you. Don't silently add statements to this list. Make a list of your own to reflect your own unique feelings and concerns:

My own feelings and concerns following the death of my spouse are:

_____
_____
_____
_____
_____
_____
_____
_____
_____

> **CIRCLE THIS**

Expressing your feelings: Talking about your feelings is important if the healing process is to begin. But some people ask themselves privately, 'How long will I want to talk about this? What is normal?' The answer is not simple. You may want to talk about your loss for a long time. You must talk about it for as long and as much as you like. Only stop when you don't want to talk anymore. For some people this might mean six months and for others two years or more.

It's often useful to go for counselling or to join a support group. Some hospitals have support groups for people who are suffering loss due to a specific cause.

For some women, writing about their feelings is the preferred form of expression. If you're so inclined, pen a few lines of poetry or prose. Kathleen Raine expressed her loss in the following poem:

Spell Against Sorrow

Who will take away
Carry away sorrow,
Bear away grief?

Talon and beak
Pluck out the heart
And the nerves of pain
Tear away grief.

For women who wish to attempt writing about their feelings, it's important to remember to not be self-conscious. Kay, 56, gives this advice:

> *'Don't think too much about how you're writing. Just express yourself, your feelings and thoughts. For me writing was useful, because it helped occupy me during the days and nights I couldn't rest or sleep. Just follow your instinct. Often I'd be writing and I'd start crying or I'd be crying and then I'd be writing. It made me feel much better.'*

Perhaps one of the following exercises will help you get started in expressing yourself on paper. Once you've begun, just follow your instinct as Kay suggests, and express your own individual needs and reactions.

> **Exercise** — **Expressing your feelings through writing**

- **Write a description of your spouse.**
Create this pen-picture as if it were for someone who had never met him. Include all aspects of his personality, character, speech, gestures, habits, appearance, intelligence, humour, preferences. Remember to include everything that made him unique.

- **Write a farewell letter to your spouse.**
In this piece, you should attempt to be thorough. It is a good-bye. Tell him what you are feeling, what you miss most, what you will always remember and cherish. Write honestly about what the relationship gave you. And how your life will forever be influenced by having known and loved him.

- **Reflect on your major feeling regarding your loss.**
Ask yourself is it loneliness, incompleteness, anger, guilt, remorse? Write as much as you can about this feeling. Explore the feeling. Don't be afraid and don't deny it.

MEETING CHALLENGES AND ANTICIPATING ANNIVERSARIES

Strangely enough, women who've lost their spouses often reveal that it is emotionally easier for them to interact with new people or friends who were not the 'couple's' friends only. One client, Kathleen, confides, *'I think I'm a visual reminder to them that one half of the couple is missing. It seems to threaten people. Maybe they fear that their own coupleness is in jeopardy.'*

Other women have reported that long-standing friends sometimes avoid mentioning their husband's name in conversation. While this may be done out of embarrassment and sensitivity for the widow's feelings, it often is experienced quite differently. Kathleen confesses when this happens, she gets angry and has been known to confront the friend. She says, *'I know it's probably done to spare my feelings, but the reverse actually happens. I feel as though they are wiping out 35 years of my life, as though it never existed.'*

Another challenge faced by women who've lost their spouse is avoiding rooms and even furniture which reminds them of their husband. Some women have reported feeling emotionally distraught when passing their husband's favorite chair. This pain may diminish with time, but if a woman's life is seriously inhibited by this behaviour she should seek professional help.

Yet another challenge is that of experiencing hallucinations. Some women say that they feel an invisible presence, see their husbands or talk to them, especially in the first year following the death. Researchers have recorded women saying that they could hear and smell their husbands. It is thought that this form of 'presence' is a product of the woman's sensory recall. And her strong feelings. These illusions can ease a woman's pain, give her reassurance and comfort her in her loneliness. She need not feel 'crazy'. Such incidents of illusions are not harmful and do not indicate any abnormality.

Anniversaries – of his birthday, your wedding day and of his death are particularly painful times. Consciously or unconsciously, a woman may experience intense sadness and grief in the days leading up to these events. It's useful to anticipate the day, by taking control of the day in advance. Make plans for the day. Visit with a friend. Make sure you are not passive in how you will spend the day. Many women have said how helpful they have found a phone call from a trusted friend or member of a support group on the day, expressing empathy for the woman on a day full of sad memories.

Above all, it's important to acknowledge the powerful feelings such days raise in a woman. Silence about these days only brings emptiness and a sense of vulnerability.

It is silence and a sense of vulnerability that mark another potential vulnerable point in a woman's life. Crimes of the heart can be committed by either a man against a woman or a woman against a man.

VULNERABLE LIFE POINT 6: HIS AND HER CRIMES OF THE HEART

'He told me he'd been with another woman...'

Twelve years ago, Louise caught a sexually transmitted disease from her husband. That was the beginning of the story. And her discovery of a secret she would never have suspected. She says,

'He told me he'd been with another woman. I believed him. But he'd lied. Years later I discovered the truth. It wasn't until I checked his pockets that the truth hit me. That was much later. Maybe eight years later. Then the man I thought I'd known for fifteen years was standing before me, admitting to me that he met men for casual sex. Worse still, what I'd found in his jacket pocket was a love letter from another man. He admitted he was in love with this man and had been seeing him for two years. I thought I was going to die! It seemed one thing losing your husband to another woman, but it was quite another thing losing him to a man.'

Louise goes on to say that her husband's behaviour made sense to her in hindsight. Little things that she'd pushed to the back of her mind over the years started to make more sense. In retrospect, she 'remembered' the sex books, magazines, toys and condoms. She 'remembered' that he had more headaches than she ever had in their relationship over the years. And she 'remembered' his chiding of her as having a 'puritanical' attitude towards sex, because she wouldn't indulge in what she considered 'kinky'. What was safely locked away in Louise's unconscious mind surfaced and became conscious once the final piece of the jigsaw was put into place.

Humiliation set in first for Louise. Other women in similar situations report a similar initial response. She thought she must be a complete failure as a woman for him to turn to men for sexual gratification. Then she went on the roller-coaster ride of feelings: shock, self-recrimination, anger and depression.

When a woman discovers her partner has been unfaithful, she feels betrayed. But when her partner has chosen another man, the rejection a woman feels is enormous.

Louise put it succinctly when she said,

'If your husband has an affair with another woman it's incredibly threatening, but you think you can compete against her. But when he's seeing another man, you simply can't do what a man does. This leaves you feeling sexually useless and helpless. The anger and depression sets in. It's very disempowering. It knocks your self-esteem terribly.'

This knocked self-esteem and the feelings of disempowerment is often reinforced by the shock, isolation and stigma of having a husband who is gay. The woman needs support and she needs to ventilate her feelings. Professional help is available and there are even support groups in some areas for women with gay or bisexual partners.

New knowledge like this may create a reaction in a woman where she believes her mind has spun out of control. She may long desperately for yesterday, only she must accept that there was no yesterday, only her perception of it.

A perception of being an observer, not a participant in life is often expressed by women who commit crimes of the heart – and pay the price through depression. Single women who have affairs with married men often feel like they are really living only 'half a life'.

BITTER-SWEET ROMANCE: LIFE AS THE 'OTHER WOMAN'

When women are feeling virtuous, they chat with each other bravely about how they wouldn't accept not being number one and philosophically and morally recoil at the thought of sharing a man with his wife. 'I would always come first', they say.

Being the other woman might be bruising to your ego and morally unsound – but a lot of women have occupied that position.

In Bruce Beresford's movie *Crimes of the Heart*, a woman returns to her family home in the small town in which she grew up. She sees her old lover, whom she left behind. He has married someone else, but within 24 hours of her arrival, he pulls up in his battered pick-up truck outside her front door. They recapture their old romance. They drink and laugh and dance in the sand beside the lake. The lovers, played by Jessica Lange and Sam Shepard, have a hunger for each other which moves beyond the erotic to the heart and soul. Their intimacy is intense. However, in the morning, the Jessica Lange character walks back alone.

Her two sisters are sitting at the kitchen table. She leans against the refrigerator and smiles at her sisters: "I was waiting for him to say 'I'll leave my wife and children: just say you'll stay with me.' 'But,' she laughs, "he didn't say it!" The man returns to his wife and children. The woman laughs at her own absurdity in expecting anything else. It is this self-mocking attitude that can turn from seemingly philosophical to very desperate in time. The desperation leads to a sense of vulnerability.

Christine was 'the other woman' for ten years. In those ten years, her feelings and attitude underwent tremendous change. She began by wondering, if he wanted her and needed her as passionately as this, how could he go back to his wife? After ten years she knew the answer. She was a fragment of his life, a bonus in his life. But she was not his life. Her lover had no strong desire – and a lot of fear of giving up the stability and convenience of marriage. She says,

> *'I experienced a lot of ambivalence. There was the pain of contradictory passions. I was his lover – and sometimes I liked that role. Did I really want to be his wife? I didn't know. What I did know was that I wanted him to leave his wife. But it became clear as the years rolled on that he had no intention of obliging me. Oh, at first there was talk about how he would ask her for a trial separation, once the kids were older. Then the oldest child had important exams, then his mother-in-law was sick and so it went on. There was never the right time. In the end, he didn't hide behind things, he simply said, 'my wife is wonderful, loyal and supportive so how can I leave her?' I guess I accepted that. But when he started the other line of 'I don't want to hurt anybody' meaning his wife, I realised it was time to end the relationship. Obviously this man could not see or understand my hurt.'*

Being involved with a married man is an unequal relationship. It's not that 'the other woman' is not first in the man's life – she might come, at best, third or fourth after wife, family and work. And then there is the humiliating enforced passivity of waiting for him to call. Remember the feeling that Dorothy Parker's heroine had in *A Telephone Call* in a previous chapter? Many 'other women' describe that same tension. Like a teenager, the woman might circle around the telephone, feeling silly, but willing it to call. Then, maybe a call – snatched moments at the beginning or end of the day. There is overwhelming sadness as well as unbearable tenderness involved in being 'the other woman'.

Thinking through to the logical consequences of such an affair is painful. Emotions take over – and often make a woman very depressed indeed. For some women, the moment of realisation is when the thought occurs to them that, no matter how passionate the affair is, it is one-sided. There is a sense of disempowerment – he will never be there when she needs him.

There are no reliable statistics in this area, but anecdotal evidence suggests that men are more emotionally dependent on their marriages than they are on their lovers. They cling tenaciously to their marriages – and mostly, feel the piquancy of bitter-sweet pain, and even a feeling of noble sacrifice in eventually giving her up. That is, unless she gives him up first.

Anne Sexton, the popular poet of the 1960s and early 1970s was familiar with life's pain. She was born Anne Grey Harvey in Newtown, Massachusetts on November 9, 1928. She belonged to the 'confessional' school of poetry, writing about mental breakdown, sex, addiction and abortion. She was an artist. And she almost certainly suffered chronic depression throughout her life. Stepping to the podium in a long dress, she would publicly read harrowing accounts of insanity and loss. And all in her throaty, classy voice. Anne Sexton knew what to think about being the other woman. She was aware of the realistic ending. She wrote a poem simply called *For My Lover, Returning to His Wife:*

> *She is all there.*
> *She was melted carefully down for you*
> *and cast up from your childhood,*
> *cast up from your own hundred favorite aggies.*
>
> *She has always been there, my darling.*
> *She is, in fact, exquisite.*
> *Fireworks in the dull middle of February*
> *and as real as a cast-iron pot.*
>
> *Let's face it, I have been momentary.*
> *A luxury. A bright red sloop in the harbor.*
> *My hair rising like smoke from the car window.*

Littleneck clams out of season.
She is more than that. She is your have to have,
has grown you your practical your tropical growth.
This is not an experiment. She is all harmony.
She sees to oars and oarlocks for the dinghy,

has placed wild flowers at the window at breakfast,
sat by the potter's wheel at midday,
set forth three children under the moon,
three cherubs drawn by Michelangelo,

done this with her legs spread out
in the terrible months in the chapel.
If you glance up, the children are there
like delicate balloons resting on the ceiling.

She has also carried each one down the hall
after supper, their heads privately bent,
two legs protesting, person to person,
her face flushed with a song and their little sleep.

I give you back your heart.
I give you permission –
for the fuse inside her, throbbing
angrily in the dirt, for the bitch in her
and the burying of her wound –
for the burying of her small red wound alive –

for the pale flickering flare under her ribs,
for the drunken sailor who waits in her left pulse,
for the mother's knee, for the stockings,
for the garter belt, for the call –

the curious call
when you will burrow in arms and breasts
and tug at the orange ribbon in her hair

and answer the call, the curious call.

She is so naked and singular.
She is the sum of yourself and your dream.
Climb her like a monument, step after step.
She is solid.

As for me, I am a watercolour.
I wash off.

Feelings and thoughts can be confused and confusing. Sorting through your feelings and learning how to think more rationally will help resolve your dilemma. Maybe Anne Sexton's thinking will make sense for you.

You may think only the good thoughts about your life as the other woman. Yet, the dark thoughts are always close by. Often thinking is very distorted for the other woman. Many of her thoughts are irrational, and her thought process can get very confused. Learning how to think more clearly, and rationally is a good strategy to adopt to help overcome a feeling of vulnerability.

Shakespeare's Hamlet, well-known for his depression, had an insight when he said, *'There is nothing either good or bad, but thinking makes it so.'*

We all have well-traversed and well-learned ways of thinking. Habitual ways of thinking may become disrupted and distorted. Our coping may be greatly impeded and our capacity to grasp the new reality is affected and consequently, our sense of vulnerability is magnified.

What you can do is to review your thinking. Perhaps you need to understand how you think. Perhaps your thinking is negative, or irrational – by reviewing and taking control, you will be in a position to make changes. When you're depressed, your thinking may not be as 'straight' as you'd like. Learning to feel better by thinking straighter is important if you're to begin regaining control over your life.

FEELING BETTER BY THINKING STRAIGHTER

Thoughts can have a profound effect on your mood. Working with thoughts has its advantages. They are always with you, so it's good to understand their impact on you. They are under your control.

Two characteristics of thoughts are worth noting.

1. Thoughts seem automatic

It's easy to take them for granted. You must learn to become aware of them, take them seriously, and, at times, work towards change

2. Thoughts cannot be observed by other people

They are private and only you will know what you think

There is a direct relationship between thoughts and feelings: how you think determines how you feel. People sometimes have negative thoughts. When things aren't going well, or you're anxious or down, then your thoughts are more likely to be illogical, and everything will seem worse than it is. Distortions in your thinking can lead to over-reaction to everyday situations.

Learn to identify your thinking habits. One way of managing your emotional reactions is by thinking 'straighter'. By changing your thoughts, you can also modify unhelpful reactions.

MENTAL RELAXATION: FEELING BETTER BY THINKING STRAIGHTER

- Whenever you have negative feelings, say a coping statement to yourself
- Back it up with constructive action
- Teach yourself to think more rationally
- Find the irrational beliefs in what you are thinking
- Practice, practice, practice, a more rational view

Mental relaxation is a technique. It is different from physical relaxation, but similar in aim because it is intended to help you feel more relaxed and comfortable. Mental relaxation means using your mind to relax your emotions. Although the technique is called relaxation, it's a very active coping skill. The activity, of course, is taking place inside your head.

The process of mental relaxation is broken down into several steps. It often helps people learning how to do mental relaxation to do it as a written exercise. An example of this form, called a Mental Relaxation Report, will be given later.

COPING WITH BAD OR NEGATIVE FEELINGS

When you find you feel bad, or down and low it's all too easy to stay with that feeling. If you do, then you'll think of how badly off you are, start feeling sorry for yourself and reinforce the original bad feeling about yourself.

You can manage these bad feelings by saying a coping statement to yourself and backing it up with some constructive action. The coping statement is a set of instructions you give to yourself, whenever you feel bad or low. When you act on these instructions as you say them to yourself, your negative feelings should lessen.

In the beginning, it helps if you write down the coping statement and carry it around with you. You'll find that when you need it most is when it can be hard to think straight or remember anything constructive. Write the coping statement on a card which you can pull out and read to yourself when you need to. Once you've used the coping statement a few times, you'll find you have learned it by heart.

Your coping statement is not a 'magic' formula. It's not like 'abracadabra'. It is important that it means something to you and that you recite it with intention and purpose.

The basic formula for a coping statement
- I expect some bad and down feelings in this situation, but I'll cope
- I won't deny my feelings, but I also won't dwell on them
- If possible, I'll do something constructive, to improve the situation
- If not, I'll do something else, pleasant or constructive, to distract me

LET'S TAKE THIS FORMULA STEP BY STEP:

'I expect some bad and down feelings in this situation, but I'll cope...'
Begin coping by reminding yourself that it's normal to have bad, down and negative feelings under certain circumstances. But then go on to remind yourself that you will cope with these feelings.

Don't expect to suddenly feel great. 'Coping' in this sense means managing or dealing with the situation. So, the statement means: 'I expect to have some normal bad and down feelings in these circumstances, but I'll manage them.'

'...*I won't try to deny my feelings, but I also won't dwell on them...*'
Sometimes people fall into the trap of saying things to themselves like: 'This is silly, I shouldn't be feeling like this', or 'It's crazy (or weak or stupid or cowardly) to feel like this. What's wrong with me?'

Trying to deny your feelings is likely to have you feeling bad about feeling bad, because you've told yourself you shouldn't be feeling bad.

Another trap is wallowing in your bad and down feelings. After an hour or day of stewing over your feelings, you will find you feel worse, but you haven't achieved anything. The dwelling and stewing hasn't taken away your feelings. The only real effect of dwelling on your negative feelings is to make you feel worse.

Of course, you have to practice not stewing on bad feelings. As you may have discovered, it is easier to tell yourself to stop stewing than to do so.

'...*if possible, I'll do something constructive to improve the siutation now...*'
Getting yourself into gear and doing something practical is the best way of stopping yourself from dwelling unnecessarily on your bad feelings. Choose something that will improve your situation directly.

Constructive action is the best antidote to dwelling and stewing. You can do something constructive about your feelings by sharing them. Or you can plan something you can do tomorrow. Or you can adopt a distraction strategy.

'...*if not, I'll do something else, pleasant or constructive, to distract me.*'
A distraction strategy is useful to block the unnecessary dwelling. Distract yourself with any activity that will occupy your mind. Choose a constructive activity like working on a hobby, or a pleasant activity, such as reading a book or socialising with a friend.

What matters is that you are occupied and not tempted to slip back into stewing over a situation about which you can do nothing.

Exercise: Putting it together

It's time to put some of what you've read together. Follow the steps set out below:

Say the coping statement to yourself
You recognise that you have a strong negative feeling, which has been triggered by something outside or inside you. You begin mental relaxation by saying the coping statement to yourself.

Back it up with constructive action
Your coping statement tells you to do something constructive to improve the situation, or if that's not possible, to distract yourself.

Teach yourself to think rationally
Saying your coping statement and backing it up with constructive action are important to do at the time you feel bad and down.

But, let's look at what you can do between your periods of feeling bad and down. You can work on thinking more rationally about problem situations you face. Your aim is to work out what your thoughts are about a situation, then test those thoughts for mistakes and irrationality, which helps you work out a more realistic way of thinking about the situation.

What is your original self-talk?
Your original self-talk refers to what is going through your mind at the time you're having the strong negative feelings. This self-talk can be in words or images, that is, what you're thinking and what you're imagining.

The idea behind mental relaxation is that your original self-talk has a major influence on your feelings. So, if your feelings are very strong, or persist for a long time, it could be because of mistakes in your self-talk. Maybe your self-talk is exaggerating your bad feelings. Your first step is to work out what your self-talk is. When you're in a situation which is likely to trigger bad and down feelings, what is your self-talk?

Imagine yourself in the trigger situation. Then imagine how you feel in that situation. Now try to work out what you were thinking or imagining while you were experiencing those bad and down feelings.

Test your self-talk for mistakes
We tend to believe our own thoughts. We are inclined to say something to ourselves and to accept it as accurate, true and realistic. However, often it isn't.

When you accept mistakes in your self-talk as though they were accurate, then those mistakes make more extra bad feelings. The situation might have made you feel bad, but your thinking mistakes will add to those bad feelings. You have to learn to identify and get rid of the mistakes.

Look at the following list of nine common thinking mistakes.

COMMON MISTAKES IN THINKING

1. Overgeneralising

This involves drawing a general conclusion on the basis of only one incident. What happens here is that you tell yourself that, if something is true in one case, it will apply to any case that is even remotely similar. However, life is rarely that simple.

2. Black and white thinking

This sort of thinking means you see things as being either/or, one extreme or the other. For instance, you tell yourself that a friendship must be very good, otherwise it is very bad. Life, in the real world, offers many shades of grey.

3. 'Who needs evidence?'

This thinking involves drawing a conclusion without any real evidence to support it, or even in the face of contradictory evidence. For instance, thinking that no-one likes you, when you have friends and you haven't asked everyone you know their feelings about you. Test yourself by asking, 'What is the real world evidence to support my conclusions in this self-talk?'

4. Looking at the world through blue glasses

This means focusing on what you think is wrong – your problems, your failures – and blowing it up out of all proportion. You ignore, belittle or discount anything that's good – your good times, your successes and achievements.

This is the flip-side to looking at the world through rose-coloured glasses. Don't distort the world in either direction.

5. Imagining the worst

This is the sort of thinking which comes from looking at the world through very deep blue glasses. It is a special case of exaggeration. Imagining the worst means assuming the worst possible outcome for an event. This is usually so exaggerated that it's highly improbable, if not impossible.

6. Taking things personally

This thinking blames yourself for everything that's wrong, even when you may not be responsible. For instance, you blame only yourself for all the problems in your relationship, although in reality, your partner contributes to them too. Remember, you don't run the whole universe. Personalising can also mean you think that everybody notices everything about you and every mistake you make – you are the centre of everybody's disapproving attention. Of course, most people are more concerned about their own problems and may not even notice yours.

7. Mistaking feelings for facts – I feel therefore I am
This thinking confuses feelings with reality. For instance, you may believe that because you feel hopeless, you are hopeless. If you feel hurt, you believe that you have been wronged. You need to recognise that feelings, no matter how real they are to you, are not objective facts.

8. Converting positives into negatives
This thinking is pessimistic and results in you becoming suspicious and cynical of people's motives. A good example is refusing to accept a compliment, by thinking 'What's she after?'. Or you may think 'he's just saying that because he knows I feel bad, but he doesn't mean it'. By doing this, you are dismissing a compliment and depriving yourself of a boost to your confidence. Remember, when you turn a positive experience into an unpleasant or neutral one by not giving yourself credit for your good points, your achievements, you prevent yourself from building self-esteem.

9. Setting unrealistic expectations
People prone to the blues tend to set higher and more unattainable goals. There is a danger in living by fixed rules. This sort of thinking ensures that you are doomed to fail in your own eyes. When you think this way, you will often say things beginning with:

- I must... (do it perfectly)
- I have to... (have a tidy desk)
- I've got to... (stick to it)
- I should... (be doing something else)
- I need... (someone to love me)

Although some of these statements may look reasonable, in context they become unreasonable. 'Should' and 'must' statements serve to remind you of what you're not doing, creating unnecessary disappointment and bad feelings.

Women who feel depressed and low are sometimes reluctant to admit that there might be any mistakes in their view of the world. They might think, 'It's really like that, it's bad and that's why I feel so bad.'

For your own sake, take a critical look at your self-talk, and save yourself from unnecessary bad and down feelings.

Learn these nine common thinking mistakes and analyze your own thinking style. Could your self-talk be more positive?

LOOK FOR UNDERLYING IRRATIONAL BELIEFS

We are not born able to think. Our thinking develops throughout life. We learn how and what to think from those around us. Sometimes, what we have learnt to think is irrational or unrealistic. There are some common irrational beliefs that most of us have been exposed to. As a result, most of us are influenced by these beliefs at different times. The trouble with these beliefs if that they are irrational. Consequently, when we allow them to influence us we are likely to feel bad and to handle life less well than we could.

Read the following irrational beliefs one at a time, pausing at each one to decide if it has influenced you.

Ten popular irrational beliefs

1. I must be loved, or at least liked, and approved by every significant person I meet.
2. If I am to be worthwhile, I must be completely competent, make no mistakes, and achieve in every possible way.
3. Some people are bad and wicked and they should be blamed and punished for this.
4. It is dreadful, nearly the end of the world, when things don't go how I'd like them to.
5. Unhappiness, including mine, is caused by factors outside my control, so I can do little about it.

6. If something might be unpleasant or frightening, I should worry about it a great deal.
7. It's easier to put off something unpleasant or difficult than it is to face up to it.
8. I need to depend on someone stronger than myself.
9. My problem(s) were caused by event(s) in my past, and that's why I have problem(s) now.
10. I should be very upset by other people's problems and difficulties.

You may recognise that you have been influenced by most of these irrational beliefs at some time. Think about which ones are influencing your current situation.

Testing your self-talk for both thinking mistakes and irrational beliefs is important. It's been found that the more you challenge your old self-talk the more effective mental relaxation is.

The thinking mistakes are errors in how you are thinking. The irrational beliefs are errors in what you are thinking. So, for the greatest positive effects, you must question your original self-talk for both style and content.

NOW PRACTISE A MORE RATIONAL VIEW

Now that you've identified any common thinking mistakes you are making and any underlying irrational beliefs that caused you to overreact to your trigger situations you're ready for the next step. Your mistaken and irrational self-talk has increased your bad and down feelings. So the question is, 'What do I say to myself instead?'

To help you plan better self-talk to use in future situations, ten rational ideas are listed below. These ideas avoid the common thinking mistakes and replace the irrational beliefs.

Ten rational ideas

1. I want to be loved or liked or approved of by some of the people in my life and I will feel disappointed when that doesn't happen. But I can cope with those feelings. I can take constructive steps to make and keep better relationships.
2. I want to do some things well, most of the time. Like everybody, I will

occasionally fail or make mistakes. If this happens and I feel bad, I can cope with that. I can take constructive steps to do better next time.
3. It is sad that some people do some bad things from time to time. But making myself upset won't change that.
4. It is disappointing when things aren't how I'd like them to be. But I can cope with that. I can take constructive steps to make things more as I would like them to be. But if I can't, it doesn't help me to exaggerate my disappointment.
5. My problem(s) may be influenced by factors outside my control, but my thoughts and actions also influence my problem(s), and they are under my control.
6. Worrying about something that might go wrong won't stop it from happening, it just makes me unhappy now. I can take constructive steps to prepare for possible problems, and that's as much as anyone can do. So I won't dwell on the future now.
7. Facing difficult situations will make me feel bad at the time, but I can cope with that. Putting off problems doesn't make them go away, or any easier to deal with. It just gives me longer to worry about them.
8. It's good to get support from others when I want it, but I need to learn to rely on myself as well.
9. My problem(s) may have started in some past events, but what keeps it (them) going now are my thoughts and actions, and they are under my control.
10. It is sad to see other people who are in trouble, but I don't help them my making myself miserable. I can cope with feeling sad. Sometimes I can take constructive steps to help them.

The numbers of the rational ideas match those of the irrational beliefs.

Read over the rational ideas that match your chosen irrational beliefs, one at a time. The aim here is for you to think differently the next time your bad feelings are triggered by a situation. After you read each of the matching rational ideas, stop and reflect on how you might apply it to your own situation.

VULNERABLE POINTS AND PROCESSES

PUTTING TOGETHER WHAT YOU'VE LEARNED

To help you master mental relaxation, look at the sample Mental Relaxation Report which appears below.

Mental Relaxation Report Form

Describe the situation that has triggered your bad feelings:

Break-up with my boyfriend

Describe your feelings:

Angry then depressed

Say the coping statement to yourself (using your feelings and situation, if you like)

I expect some bad feelings in this situation, but I'll cope

What constructive steps did you take or have you planned?

Lessen my depression with a coping statement and some distracting activities

What is your original self-talk in the situation?

I can never have a good relationship.
I'm always going to be haunted by what happened.
I'll never feel OK about a relationship again.

Which common thinking mistakes can you find in your self-talk?
(Just list the number/s)   *1, 3, 5*

Which irrational belief/s seem to be influencing your original reaction?
(Just list the number/s)   *4, 5*

Now practise the matching rational idea/s trying to apply it/them to your situation.

Now it's time to complete you own Mental Relaxation Report Form . . .

| Exercise | Mental relaxation report |

Start learning how to use mental relaxation now. On the blank Report Form, write a brief description of the situation that involves negative feelings. List the feelings.

If you can't find an apparent trigger for your bad feelings, maybe it's because you've been doing too much dwelling on your bad feelings themselves. If that's the case, record on your Report Form something like, 'Thinking about how dreadful my experience at work was.'

Mental Relaxation Report Form

Describe the situation that has triggered your bad feelings:

_____
_____
_____
_____

Describe your feelings:

_____
_____
_____
_____

Say the coping statement to yourself (use your feelings and situation, if you like)

_____
_____
_____
_____

What constructive steps did you take or have you planned?

_____
_____
_____
_____

What is your original self-talk in the situation?

_____
_____
_____
_____

Which common thinking mistakes can you find in your self-talk?
(Just list the number/s) _____

Which irrational belief/s seem to be influencing your original reaction?
(Just list the number/s) _____

Practice the matching rational idea/s trying to apply it/them to your situation.

By now you should have worked through one complete example of mental relaxation. You will only get the benefit it has to offer if you do it and don't just read it. After you've tried one example for yourself, try a couple more while it's fresh in your mind. You will find that you can master the procedure more easily initially if you do it in writing. It's something you'll need to do over and over again. You are often setting out to change some entrenched thinking habits. You need to be persistent.

Whenever you feel bad and down, use the mental relaxation to help yourself feel less bad and prompt yourself to do something constructive. You will find it a useful coping skill.

(Adapted from *Mental Relaxation*, Montgomery and Morris, 1989)

TEST YOUR KNOWLEDGE OF THINKING MISTAKES OR DISTORTIONS

Now you're ready to do a Thinking Distortions quiz. Test yourself on the common mistakes in thinking you can make. Remember the nine mistakes in thinking we covered earlier – overgeneralising, black and white thinking, 'who needs evidence?', looking at the world through blue glasses, imagining the worst, taking things personally, mistaking feelings for facts, converting positives into negatives and setting unrealistic expectations.

Exercise: Thinking distortions quiz

There are thinking distortions in each of the following situations.
- Underline the key words which point to the thinking mistake
- Record which thinking distortion is operating.

1. Jemima is about to go for a job interview. She thinks to herself, 'This is my last chance. If I don't get this job, then it shows that I'm a failure'
   Distortion _____

2. When Kerry arrives at work one morning, one of her colleagues walks past and simply grunts at her. Kerry thinks, 'No one says hello to me anymore'
   Distortion _____

3. Diana's friends tell her how much they admire her for the ungrudging efforts she put into caring for her dying father. She replies, 'Oh, anyone could have done it'
   Distortion _____

4. Barbara is the first female executive in her company. She sits in the boardroom and thinks, 'I should be happy all the time. I have no right to ever feel down'
   Distortion _____

5. Erica is about to introduce a new business associate to a group of colleagues, but forgets his name. She thinks, 'How embarrassing. I wish I could just disappear. I'll never be able to face anyone again. I'll never get over this'
   Distortion _____

6. The manager returns a report which Lee-anne has prepared. He commented that it was a good piece of work, but that there were a few spelling mistakes which needed to be corrected. Lee-anne thinks, 'He must think I'm stupid for not being able to spell. He thinks I've given him a bad report'
   Distortion _____

7. Catherine is talking with some of her daughter's friends. She thinks 'That's the third time they've interrupted me. Obviously they're bored with me and my conversation. I must be a real dull person'
   Distortion _____

8. Julia is about to go to a party, but she gets cold feet. She thinks, 'I feel so dull and uninteresting. I won't know what to say to anyone'
   Distortion _____

9. Angie is at a busy diner with a friend. The waitress is giving them bad service. She thinks, 'I must have offended her somehow'
   Distortion _____

Note: Answers to the quiz follow, but don't peek!

Answers to the quiz
1. Black and white thinking
2. Overgeneralizsing
3. Converting positives into negatives
4. Setting unrealistic expectations
5. Imagining the worst
6. Looking at the world through blue glasses
7. 'Who needs evidence?'
8. Mistaking feelings for facts
9. Taking things personally

(Adapted from *Thinking Distortions Quiz*, Tanner and Ball, 1989)

10

TAKING CONTROL OF YOUR LIFE

Action is the antidote to despair.

JOAN BAEZ

The best way to overcome your depression is to recognise your vulnerability and then the initiative to regain control. Now that you've read about depression and its causes and heard from other women, it's over to you. You've done the exercises and tasks along the way and you have learned some new strategies. You are the only one who can make sense of your experience of depression and learn what helps you. Knowing how to manage your low feelings is very empowering.

You might decide to seek the assistance of professionals or you might decide to use some self-help strategies which have helped other women. Read all the information, study the exercises, try them and you'll discover which of them work best for you. By doing so, you're observing Joan Baez's words: *'Action is the antidote to despair'*.

Helping professionals are a source of support and confidence. Maybe you think you need to see a therapist or counsellor – someone to whom you can ventilate your feelings and someone in whom you can confide. For a long time now, helping professionals have said that the ability to allow your real self to be known to at least one other person is a pre-requisite for a healthy personality. In fact, studies have demonstrated that not having a confiding relationship makes you more vulnerable to emotional problems, like depression. So confiding is good for your immune system and your body and your emotions and soul.

The person in whom you confide need not be a professional. Some women have found support and confidence in their family members, friends, colleagues and formal support groups.

One woman, Tamara, 29 says,

> 'You just need to tell one other person how miserable you feel. And then you start feeling better. It's not that you expect them to do anything, just to listen and try to understand, that's enough. I use a good friend for this – she's warm, she's understanding and most of all, she doesn't judge me. She's really in tune with me.'

Finding a support group is one thing you can do. Becoming a member of a group can mean finding other people who understand you. You can also find new friends in such groups. Some people find support groups provide them with a strong feeling of support and help them keep their vulnerability to the blues at bay. Check your newspaper for support groups or ask a counsellor.

Other people, like Tamara, find that seeking out support from one or more friends is what they need to help them out of their blues. Psychologically, the act of confiding in another human being lessens your load and lightens your mood. Expressions such as 'getting it off your chest' and 'no man (or woman) is an island' are evidence of the need we humans have to confide in others.

Here are some comments women have made about what they look for and need when it comes to support and confidence in the face of their depression:

'You need someone to affirm you and your strengths'

'Treating me with humour and respect – validating me, that's what it's all about'

'I know that I need someone to empathise with me, not sympathise. I want them to say "Gee, it's rough for you, I can understand what you're going through"'

'When I've got the blues, I want a person or people around me to bring me out of myself – you know, to help me to celebrate life again, sing, dance, have fun again'

'I have to trust the person and they have to respect me and my feelings. They have to be open-minded, so I can feel I can be myself and not scare them away'

'It helps me if I can have a trusted person monitor me when I'm depressed, usually because I can't do it well myself when I'm feeling low'

'If you've got the blues you need people to validate you – help you to believe in yourself and to encourage your dreams and hopes'

'I look for someone who can accept me and not be judgemental. Someone who can feel along with me and at the same time, offer me encouragement and support to work myself out of the blues'

Look at the following exercise. It makes you think about what you want when you're feeling vulnerable.

Exercise: What do you want from your support system?

Tick those things which you want from your support system:

- ☐ Someone to talk to
- ☐ Understanding
- ☐ Acceptance
- ☐ Someone who will listen
- ☐ Empathy
- ☐ Sharing
- ☐ Companionship
- ☐ Caring
- ☐ Time
- ☐ Activities
- ☐ Diversion
- ☐ Monitoring

Sometimes people who are vulnerable to depression have a hard time making and keeping friends. One reason for this is because they may have low self-esteem. Another reason is because they have a hard time with reaching out to others. Yet another reason is because they have poor social skills. Working on your self-esteem and boosting your self-confidence means that you will feel more comfortable about yourself and reaching out to others. Your social skills will be improved.

Go back and read over the chapters on self-esteem and communication skills. And work on your skills. Practise, practise, practise.

Now you can think of specific people to support you.

Exercise: Supportive people I know

List three people who you feel you can reach out to for support and confidence when you've got the blues:

1. _____
2. _____
3. _____

If you can't think of three people, then your task is to start building your personal support network. Develop your network to at least three people, and more if you can.

One good way of building your support network is by becoming active, joining organisations and offering your services. For instance, you can consult your local paper to see if there are community activities you can join or hook into a special interest group. Consider doing some volunteer work. Many people find volunteer work makes them feel much better, because they are doing something for others. It makes them feel worthwhile.

Don't despair if these suggestions are not for you. Research evidence suggests that support and confiding can be much more individual and personal for some people. Confiding, for instance, can be effective even when it is not spoken. Also, the beneficial effects of confiding may extend to any act of confiding, for example, religious confession and even keeping a diary. For people with a creative streak, the act of writing or painting or any other creative activity, may serve the same function.

The important thing to remember, is that you need to feel like you can unload some of those unpleasant feelings associated with your feelings of vulnerability.

Remember this: Support and confiding is good for your body and soul.

And now for some self-help strategies...

When you're down, it can be hard to make a start. This exercise helps a woman believe she has the ability to take responsibility for making her life work. She can blossom into the fullness of life and what it has to offer.

Exercise: Mirror, Mirror On the Wall

Step one
Find the biggest mirror you can and look at your reflection straight in the eye.

Step two
Using your name, tell yourself exactly what you are going to do to feel better today.

Step three
Then tell the person you see in the mirror that you care enough about her to take that first step. You care enough to put the work in and to take the responsibility to overcome your blues. Say something like: 'Linda, I care about you and promise to look after you, believe in you and work towards making you feel better about yourself and the world around you'.

Step four
Remind yourself that every day when you look in the mirror to put on your make-up, brush your teeth, you are going to see yourself in the eye. So you'll need to work hard to keep that promise to yourself.

And did you know that twenty years ago researchers discovered that exercise helps lift your mood?

CIRCLE THIS – RELAXATION THROUGH EXERCISE

Aerobic exercise increases oxygen to your brain. It makes you feel more alert and increases your ability to concentrate. Try to exercise aerobically on a regular basis. As your level of fitness increases, so does your new-found energy – and good feelings about yourself. Exercise helps you develop a new image of yourself – one that is healthy. You might find yourself eating more healthy foods – and a changed sleeping pattern. Many women report not requiring anywhere near the amount of sleep they once did.

WHY NOT WALK YOUR BLUES AWAY?

Doing something physical helps you to divert your energy. Walk off that negative! But you have to walk vigorously – because the physical activity takes your focus away from the feelings that are building tension.

Try complementing your exercise program by learning to deep breathe – and notice the difference...

Remember this: Try a deep breathing technique – it's good for you.

This deep breathing technique complements your exercise program. It helps you achieve a state of mental relaxation. This is a two-step procedure. First, as you breathe in deeply, concentrate totally on your breath and imagine 'holding on' as you clear your mind of all thoughts and concerns. The 'letting go' action is to breathe out deeply. Go on, expel all the air in your lungs and let go of all your thoughts, concerns and pressures.

Deep breathing allows your body to re-energise. Some women say that they find it helpful to have a mantra (a sound that has no specific meaning – only a pleasant sound to you) – and silently repeat over and over as they breathe in and out – releasing all their tension.

Or try to repeat mentally to yourself a positive phrase that helps you feel better – and one that helps you deal with a stressful situation, for example, 'I can cope with my life by taking one day at a time'

And don't forget about affirmation and your imagination. Try doing the following exercise.

Exercise Affirmation and visualisation

The repetition of positive self-statements (affirmations) is a powerful tool for changing people's depressive thoughts. 'Control one's thoughts and effects are also controlled'. Follow these guiding principles:

1. **Visualise** your ability to control your own life
2. **Visualise** that which you want to happen
3. **Affirm** yourself and hold a positive image of your actualised desire in your mind – never mind that it hasn't happened yet – just keep your positive image in mind

Believe that you attract what you affirm – because like attracts like.

Develop a positive spiritual self-concept – affirm your place in the world – and affirm all life and existence:

Affirm 'I am open and receptive to the inflow and the outpouring of all there is in the universal, creative force'

Affirm 'I keep my thoughts centreed on those things that I want to see in my life'

Affirmations should be repeated at regular intervals.

Remember, everything must be imaged or imagined in order for it to happen – everything is first invisible to the eye. But with repetition – and belief in your heart and mind – you can create reality from your positive imagery. Don't say, 'I would like to have', but rather 'It is already mine'.

And now for the power of visual imagery. Many women have found the use of visual imagery to be very empowering.

Exercise Visual imagery

Visual exercises are a source of relaxation and energy renewal.

Surrender yourself to the experience. When you're depressed the experience can feel like living through the 'dark night of the soul', – surrender to a sensation that can bring unimaginable peace and stillness – and by doing so, learn that surrender is a personal giving up that is more than giving in. It is a letting go in the most profound sense.

References to light as a healing quality are common to most major religions and philosophies. Some scientists believe that light is a universal healing energy – allowing for a built-in capacity for health.

Don't force yourself to experience a light vision – instead, put yourself into a receptive frame of mind – make yourself available for the experience – as light visions are more likely to be experienced when the mind is empty of all purpose.

Exercise 1: Preparing Yourself
Close your eyes and take several slow, very deep breaths, breathing from your abdomen. With each inhalation, imagine that energy is being taken in from the universe. With each exhalation, imagine the entire body becoming more and more relaxed.

Exercise 2: Breathing Light
Now imagine that the inside of your body, from your centre out, is becoming brighter and brighter, radiant and illuminated. Allow yourself to enjoy this feeling for several moments. You are relaxed and full of energy. Open your eyes.

Exercise 3: Expanding Auras
Now imagine that a thin aura of light surrounds your entire body. It can be any colour you wish it to be. With each exhalation of breath, imagine this aura becoming brighter and brighter, more and more colourful, extending out from the body further and further. Imagine the aura filling the space around you, and extending out as far as you want it to reach.

Allow yourself to enjoy this experience for several moments.

You are now relaxed and full of energy.

Open your eyes.

There are variations on the theme. Some women may find using musical themes and metaphors useful.

The following exercises help you release your musicality and poetry.

Exercise: Imaging with music

Musical sound has been used as a healing medium over time in many cultures.

Listen to soothing music of your choice and conjure up the inner pictures the music brings to you. Day-dreamed images to music help deepen our self-discovery – and clarify our unique personal identity. Remember, the music must be something with which you can identify. Something which stirs you. This will be different for each woman. Some women might have an affinity with classical music, while others may find listening to the blues very consoling.

And now for a poetic journey through the use of psychosynthesis...

Roberto Assogioli developed an imagery therapy called psychosynthesis, designed to develop and increase personal and spiritual well-being. 'The Blossoming of the Rose' is one imagery journey a depressed person might take to facilitate further awareness about herself.

The words can be read to you or you can tape-record them and listen to the tape.

Exercise: Psychosynthesis

Sit quietly, your hands resting in your lap, much as you do in meditation. You are going on an imagery journey into the self.

Imagine you are looking at a rosebush. Visualise one stem with a rosebud and leaves. The sepals are closed and the bud appears to be green. At the very top, the tip of the bud can be seen. Visualise this vividly, holding the image clearly in your mind.

Now watch while the green sepals start to separate slowly one by one, their points turning slowly outward revealing the coloured petals which remain closed. The sepals continue to open until all of the tender bud can be seen.

Now the petals follow suit, slowly separating until a full-blown rose is in view.

At this stage, smell the perfume of the rose, inhaling its delicate, delicious, sweet scent with delight.

Now expand your visualisation to include the entire rosebush. Imagine that the life force that arises from the roots to the blossom causes the process of opening.

Finally, identify yourself with the rose itself. Symbolically, you are this rose.

In Assogioli's words: 'The same life that animates the universe and has created the miracle of the rose is producing in us alike, an even greater miracle – the awakening and development of our spiritual being and that which radiates from it.'

Open your eyes when you feel comfortable. Think about your reactions – ponder your creative, inner power. You have activated the inner flowering of your very being.

OTHER STRATEGIES

And now for some fun strategies for dealing with your blues...

Float a balloon

Imagine a negative thought being tied to a balloon. It's a symbol. You could even see it written on the balloon. Picture in your mind the balloon being released into the sky. Watch it get higher and higher. Watch it get smaller and smaller. Watch it disappear into a speck. The balloon, with your negative thought tied to it, eventually fades from view completely.

This helps you mentally distance yourself from the negative.

Sink the stone
This is a similar technique to floating the balloon – but in a different direction. You can mentally attach a negative thought to a stone and imagine tossing it into the deepest part of a stream – or perhaps the ocean. Watch as the stone sinks slowly until it comes to rest on the bottom of the ocean or lake.

Release fear, anxiety, doubts and guilt. Sink fear, anxiety, doubts and guilt.

Wear a protective helmet
Imagine putting on an imaginary helmet which protects you from negatives! While you wear this helmet, you can tell yourself that negatives simply bounce off – not influencing you at all! Tell yourself that negatives in your mind evaporate. The helmet is not real, but then again maybe neither are your fears and concerns.

Write out and dispose
Write out the details of the negative affecting you – and then crumple up the paper with absolute delight! Go on – tear it to pieces before throwing it out. Think about the letter written in anger, and not sent. It's a way of releasing a negative, without attracting any consequences!

Remember the saying: 'The pen is mightier than the sword'

Return to sender
Think of the old Elvis Presley song – and mentally see the negative leaving you. Picture the negative words on a card with a return stamp on it – and see it making its way back to the sender.

SOME QUICK SELF-HELP STRATEGIES...

- Read some inspirational literature – even one paragraph
- Look at a photo or picture that gives you pleasure
- Listen to some favourite music
- Selecting a memory from a prepared list of good moments. Think of the times that gave you a good feeling. Recall one such event and the feeling at the time.

It's time to put things into perspective. A woman must expect that her mood will fluctuate from time to time. There will be times when you'll feel up and times when you'll feel down – that's simply part of being human. But, you should have a lot of skills that you can use to prevent that vulnerable feeling taking over your life. You've got skills to help yourself feel better if depression does creep in. Below, you'll find a checklist to review:

MAINTAINING YOUR GAINS CHECKLIST

- Give yourself credit
- Recognise and make room for the high points – the pleasurable activities and achievements in your life
- Break old habits of negative thinking
- Think more realistically
- Relax
- Set goals and priorities
- Reward yourself for mastering plans and activities
- Be positive
- Find support and a confidante
- Respect yourself
- Communicate your thoughts and feelings
- Assert yourself

You may have reached this point and wondered if you can really be positive in your thinking.

BEING POSITIVE

If you've thought negatively for a long while, then it is hard to generate positive thoughts. Look at the negative thoughts listed below and check out the corresponding more helpful, alternative ways of viewing the situation.

Negative thoughts	Helpful thoughts
I can't cope	It feels terrible, but I am hanging on in there and I can overcome it
What's the point of trying?	If I don't try, I'll never know
I can't do it	It seems hard, but I'll find out more if I try. The more I do, the easier it will get.

What if I lose control?	If I get emotional, it's not the end of the world. After all, everyone gets upset sometimes.
I can't seem to concentrate	If I relax, my concentration will improve.

The more you repeat positive helpful thoughts to yourself the more you'll believe them and the more automatic they'll become. Motivate yourself by thinking of the benefits of a particular activity that you're finding difficult to get started.

Remember that self-doubt and self-criticism prevent you from achieving goals. They rob you of the confidence required to initiate activities and make changes in your life. You need to dispute any self-doubts. Activate thoughts that give you reassurance and confidence.

LEARN TO QUESTION YOUR THINKING

Make your thinking more effective in dealing with your stresses and strains by asking yourself these questions:

- How do I know that what I'm thinking is true?
- Are my thoughts helping me to achieve my goals?
- Are my thoughts helping me in my relationships with others?
- Is my thinking helping me feel good about myself?
- Is there another way I could think about this?
- What benefits are there in adopting another viewpoint?

BE YOUR OWN PERSON

Take a good look at all your gains. Be determined to maintain them. Work hard to understand yourself and what makes you feel vulnerable.

Think back to your Bill of Assertive Rights. You have the right to be your own person. Protect your individuality by determining which goals are appropriate and achievable for you. Setting and achieving your own goals is empowering. Managing your depression is empowering. Never giving up is empowering.

Managing your vulnerability becomes easier when you understand you need to make changes in your thinking and this will lead to changes in what you do. In the first chapter you were introduced to the idea of the relationship between your thoughts, feelings and behaviour and events in your life. Always keep that idea with you.

Each exercise and task you've completed in this book has empowered you. You've developed a range of new skills. Give yourself credit for having achieved so much. You've chosen to take control of your life. You've chosen growth over defeat. You've enhanced your well-being.

CODA

HOPE – THE LEGACY OF PANDORA

Pandora, Greek myth's Eve, was given a mysterious box by the gods. She was told never to open it. Tempted, one day, she lifted the lid and loosed into the world all the evils known. But she closed the box just in time to save an antidote: hope.

Opening up Pandora's Box and using the power of hope in your life is nurturing and empowering.

Michael D. Yapko, PhD, a therapist and writer, speaks of administering a dose of hope by encouraging his depressed patients to think about what can be, not just about what has been. 'Hopefulness is lifesaving,' he says, 'Learning to think in terms of positive possibilities is vital to defeating depression'.

CIRCLE THIS

Know the expression 'hope springs eternal'? One psychologist had proved this in his studies. Hope can be a balm, even when medicine seems helpless. Consider the plight of young victims of spinal cord injuries, paralysed for life. Timothy Elliott, PhD, interviewed 57 of these patients in rehabilitation. The most hopeful patients proved to be the least depressed. They had also managed to gain more mobility and were more likely to be active sexually and socially.

He also interviewed the nurses and found that in a ward where the burnout rate is high, the most hopeful nurses were not as drained as less hopeful ones, by the emotionally involving and draining work. It seems that for the hopeful nurses, their job gave them a sense of personal accomplishment, a meaning in their lives expressed through caring for others.

Elliott reflects, 'Hope is not just a buoyant optimism, but a sense that there is a meaning to what you do, that even the little things you do in a day make sense in terms of your larger life goals.'

Therein lies hope's ultimate power: making sense of seemingly unbearable and hopeless situations.

In the words of Vaclav Havel, the Czechoslovakian playwright and Nobel Laureate: 'Hope is an orientation of the spirit, an orientation of the heart. It is...the certainty that something makes sense, regardless of how it turns out.'

Hope is a powerful word. It is a powerful phenomenon. It is, as Vaclav Havel suggests, an orientation of the spirit and the heart – knowing that meaning can be found and life can be rewarding.

The Eve in everywoman can be transformed into the Pandora in us all. The story tells us that woman's curse began in the Garden of Eden. Eve was tempted by the serpent. She tempted Adam. And then God said: *'I will greatly multiply thy sorrow and thy conception; in sorrow thou shalt bring forth children; and thy desire shall be to thy husband, and he shall rule over thee.'* So woman has inherited the curse of Eve.

However, the myth of the goddess Pandora seeks to restore some power to women. Originally, Pandora was a goddess who held a honey vase from which she poured all good things. Not a box full of ills. Pandora, in the original texts, was called the 'All-giver' and the 'sender-forth-of-all-gifts'. In time, this changed and Pandora became the Eve figure who brought evil into the world. The Greek poet Hesiod, recorded the story of Pandora.

The story of Pandora follows.

'The first woman was called Pandora and she was fashioned from clay by the smith god Hephaistos. She was made in Heaven, every god contributing something to perfect her. Athena gave her life, Aphrodite granted her beauty. Mercury provided her with persuasion, Apollo with music and quick-witted Hermes taught her guile. Equipped with these qualities and charm, she was conveyed to Earth and presented to Epimetheus, the brother of the Titan Prometheus. Epimetheus, struck by Pandora's beauty, accepted her and the dowry of a sealed vase. Zeus had unfinished business with Prometheus, whom

CODA

be blamed for stealing fire from the heavens and giving it to humanity. Ignoring the warnings of Prometheus about Zeus' gift of Pandora, Epimetheus made her his wife. Pandora was cautioned to not open the vase, for if she did, she would loose great troubles into the world. One day, seized by curiosity, she began to finger the jar. She resolved to look inside and with some difficulty opened the tight lid.

Demons and devils flew from the vase and trembling, Pandora dropped the vase. She knew she had been tricked. Just as she began to despair, she heard a woman's voice urging her to empty the vase. In a trance, Pandora lifted the vase once more and poured from it the last vestiges of its contents. Suddenly, she became aware of a sweet scent and an ethereal form flew from the vase and circled her.

It called to her 'I am Hope'. Hope told Pandora she would alleviate the ills that Zeus had set upon the earth. And with that, Hope flew out of the window on her mission of faith and healing. Hope was sent so that hope would never entirely leave us.'

The myth of Pandora letting Hope escape into the world is a positive and empowering one. Her legacy means all women have access to an inner resource – one that offers so much positive energy and promise.

NOTES